Books should be returned to the SDH Library on or before
the date stamped above unless a renewal has been arranged

Salisbury District Hospital Library

Telephone: Salisbury (01722) 336262 extn. 4432 / 33
Out of hours answer machine in operation

Psychology in Diabetes Care

Diabetes

dp

in Practice

Other titles in the Wiley Diabetes in Practice Series

Obesity and Diabetes
Edited by Anthony Barnett and Sudhesh Kumar
0470848987

Prevention of Type 2 Diabetes
Edited by Manfred Ganz
0470857331

Diabetes - Chronic Complications Second Edition
Edited by Kenneth Shaw and Michael Cummings
0470865972

The Metabolic Syndrome
Edited by Christopher Byrne and Sarah Wild
0470025115

Exercise and Sport in Diabetes Second Edition
Edited by Dinesh Nagi
047002206X

Diabetic Cardiology
Edited by B. Miles Fisher and John McMurray
0470862041

Diabetic Nephropathy
Edited by Christoph Hasslacher
0471489921

The Foot in Diabetes Fourth Edition
Edited by Andrew J. M. Boulton, Peter R. Cavanagh and Gerry Rayman
0470015047

Nutritional Management of Diabetes Mellitus
Edited by Gary Frost, Anne Dornhorst and Robert Moses
0471497517

Hypoglycaemia in Clinical Diabetes
Edited by Brian M. Frier and B. Miles Fisher
0471982644

Diabetes in Pregnancy: An International Approach to Diagnosis and Management
Edited by Anne Dornhorst and David R. Hadden
047196204X

Childhood and Adolescent Diabetes
Edited by Simon Court and Bill Lamb
0471970034

Psychology in Diabetes Care

Second Edition

Editors

Frank J. Snoek

VU University Medical Centre, Amsterdam, The Netherlands

and

T. Chas Skinner

University of Southampton, UK

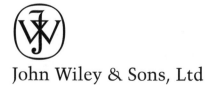

John Wiley & Sons, Ltd

Copyright © 2005   John Wiley & Sons Ltd, The Atrium, Southern Gate, Chichester,
West Sussex PO19 8SQ, England

Telephone   (+44) 1243 779777

Email (for orders and customer service enquiries): cs-books@wiley.co.uk
Visit our Home Page on www.wileyeurope.com or www.wiley.com

Other Wiley Editorial Offices

John Wiley & Sons Inc., 111 River Street, Hoboken, NJ 07030, USA

Jossey-Bass, 989 Market Street, San Francisco, CA 94103-1741, USA

Wiley-VCH Verlag GmbH, Boschstr. 12, D-69469 Weinheim, Germany

John Wiley & Sons Australia Ltd, 42 McDougall Street, Milton, Queensland 4064, Australia

John Wiley & Sons (Asia) Pte Ltd, 2 Clementi Loop #02-01, Jin Xing Distripark, Singapore 129809

John Wiley & Sons Canada Ltd, 22 Worcester Road, Etobicoke, Ontario, Canada M9W 1L1

British Library Cataloguing in Publication Data

A catalogue record for this book is available from the British Library

ISBN-13 978-0-470-02384-8
ISBN-10 0-470-02384-8

Typeset in 10.5/13pt Times by Thomson Press (India) Limited, New Delhi
Printed and bound in Great Britain by Antony Rowe Ltd, Chippenham, Wiltshire
This book is printed on acid-free paper responsibly manufactured from sustainable forestry
in which at least two trees are planted for each one used for paper production.

Contents

Foreword to the First Edition

Diabetes is a very human condition. Even to those of us with many years of clinical practice in diabetes, the infinite diversity of individual response to diabetes is a constant source of amazement but also professional enhancement. People are different and behave differently, and often unexpectedly. This is what makes involvement in diabetes care such a three-dimensional experience. Diabetes and its consequences have a fundamental physical basis, but these are deeply intertwined with complex psychosocial issues. Such interrelationships are considerable: sometimes subtle; sometimes overwhelming.

Awareness of these issues is crucial to enabling people with diabetes to lead a healthy and fulfilled life. Empathy and appreciation of the psycho-social needs of patients are essential requirements for those involved in diabetes care, and indeed most do seem to acquire that intuitive understanding of patient–professional relationships so fundamental to good clinical care. However, the world of psychology has progressed; much more is known and the evidence base of psychological management in diabetes care is becoming clearer.

Despite the widespread and increasing prevalence of diabetes in the population, the diagnosis at a personal level can still be a considerable shock and source of distress to the individual and family concerned. Suddenly a label is applied that seemingly sets them aside from others, that invokes dire consequences to both current well-being and to future health. Such initial fears and misgivings may result from misunderstandings and ignorant, albeit well intentioned, advice from others. The misguided term 'mild diabetes' may be used inappropriately to allay fears and anxieties, but in so doing it undermines the essential need to manage diabetes with due consideration and respect.

Recent published studies and clinical experience indicate that future prospects for people with diabetes should be very positive and encouraging, but despite the substantial improvements in treatments and technology a demanding daily discipline is still required.

Realistic information and education needs to be very much geared to the individual, taking into account the very diversity of such individual needs and perspectives. Necessary messages should be understood, but balancing the immediate influences on quality of life with longer term objectives on future health. Living with diabetes is a lifelong educational exercise and a similar experience for those involved in diabetes care. No amount of theoretical knowledge can match this constant learning through daily encounters with diabetes, but it is this experience that can be used to interpret and reassure. It is about achieving the right balance, and for this psychological awareness is essential.

Although the concept of a specific diabetes personality has been irrevocably refuted, diabetes will inevitably affect individuals emotionally in different ways. Both at diagnosis and in subsequent years a complex interaction between the physical consequences of diabetes and its psychological demands is constantly contributing to the vicissitudes of diabetes well-being. Even the term 'diabetes control' carries psychological undertones, but it is the term we use most frequently. Poor control may refer to inadequate achievement of good blood glucose levels, but it will also contribute to poor quality of life and often loss of personal confidence. It is the model of a vicious cycle. In contrast, for others, particularly those with type 2 diabetes, the 'silent' nature of the condition can be deceptive and deflect away from the need to maintain discipline and diligence.

Steering the narrow gap between Scylla and Charybdis is never easy, but there are now many new aids to assist the person with diabetes along the right pathway. No longer are treatments so rigid and set in tablets of stone; improved education and understanding do offer more flexibility adapted to the individual's needs.

The person with diabetes should equally contribute to discussions and decisions concerning care and best treatment, fully informed and in collaboration with the clinician. Understanding the psychosocial issues of this partnership is fundamental to success. The expert and well respected contributors to this book offer a valuable and necessary insight into the interaction between psychology and diabetes care, and in so doing provide guidance on psychological interventions to further minimize the daily demands of living with diabetes.

Professor Ken M. Shaw
March 2000

Preface to the First Edition

Psychosocial issues are increasingly recognized as being of primary importance in diabetes care. This is illustrated by the burgeoning number of publications on behavioural and social issues in both psychological and medical journals. In addition, an increasing number of international conferences and symposia on diabetes are beginning to address cognitive, emotional and behavioural issues surrounding diabetes, its complications and management. With this growing awareness of the importance of psychology in diabetes care, health care professionals experience an increasing need for easily accessible background information and practical guidelines on behavioural issues. However, only a handful of books are available for clinicians who wish to know what to do about the psychological aspects of diabetes care, from supporting patients and families coping with diagnosis and following the treatment regimen, through to complex psychological problems such as the diagnosis and management of depression and eating disorders. These are the issues this book hopes to begin to address. It seeks to bridge the gap between psychological research on the self-care and management of diabetes and the delivery of care and services provided by the diabetes care team. As such, this book is seen as an accompaniment to Clare Bradley's *Handbook of Psychology and Diabetes* (1994), which focuses on psychological assessment in diabetes. The content of this book is targeted at all individuals involved in the delivery of diabetes, including our fellow psychologists.

When considering who to ask to contribute to this book, we were acutely aware of two groups of psychologists. The largest and most well established group is the Council of Behavioural Medicine and Psychology of the American Diabetes Association (ADA). To date, these North American behavioural scientists have generated the overwhelming majority of psychological research and publications, and have compiled an excellent how-to do-it book under the editorship of Barbara Anderson and Richard Rubin (1996). Fortunately, we can see steadily increasing European work in this field, facilitated by the EASD Study Group, Psychosocial Aspects of Diabetes (PSAD). This group continues to develop and bring a distinctly European perspective to the psychology of diabetes care. Therefore, when seeking contributors for this compilation, we have endeavoured to reflect the work of both groups of researchers, thereby offering a true international perspective on psychology in diabetes care.

This book also seeks to provide a broad, evidence-based approach to behavioural intervention in diabetes care. Based on reviews of empirical and theoretical work, each chapter will make practical recommendations for diabetes care provision and future research. The authors of the nine chapters were asked to explore different approaches to intervention with children, adolescents and adults with diabetes. The first chapter is by Barbara Anderson and Julienne Brackett (USA), on diabetes during childhood, addressing developmental and family issues. Chas Skinner, Sue Chanon, Lesley Howells and Adele McEvilly (UK) then discuss the abundance of psychological literature on adolescents with diabetes, with special reference to the beliefs and attitudes of adolescents with diabetes and how these affect their self-care behaviours. Research on the psychological impact of pregnancy in diabetes is reviewed in Chapter 3 by Frank Snoek (The Netherlands), with special focus on pre-conception counselling programmes. In Chapter 4, a truly international group of authors from the USA (Bob Anderson and Martha Funnell), Sweden (Anita Carlson and Nuha Saleh-Stattin) and the UK (Sue Cradock and Chas Skinner) discusses the background and implications of the empowerment approach to diabetes education and self-management, taking into account ethnic and cultural factors. The rich potential of motivational interviewing as a vehicle for behaviour change in diabetes patients is reviewed by Yvonne Doherty, Peter James and Sue Roberts (UK) in Chapter 5. This clearly sets the stage for the Chapter by Russell Glasgow and Elizabeth Eakins (USA) on medical office-based interventions and how these can significantly contribute to the behaviour change process in diabetes. Chapters 7 and 8 expand on two different psychoeducational group programmes that were developed specifically for diabetes patients: Blood Glucose Awareness Training (BGAT), by Linda Gonder-Frederick, Daniel Cox, William Clarke and Diana Julian (USA), and Cognitive–Behavioural Group Training (CBGT), by Nicole van der Ven, Marlène Chatrou and Frank Snoek (The Netherlands). The last chapter, by Richard Rubin (USA), building on rich experience as a psychologist involved in diabetes care, reviews the indications and benefits of psychotherapy and counselling in diabetes, with reference to adaptional problems, depression, anxiety and eating disorders.

In conclusion, this book offers a comprehensive summary of current psychological knowledge and thought as it relates to the delivery of diabetes care and how to support professionals and individuals with diabetes to achieve their goals. We hope this book is a worthy start to this endeavour. Albeit incomplete, we sincerely hope you will find it informative, that it helps you reflect on your practice, whatever your professional role, and that it enables you to develop a more thoughtful approach to those individuals you are striving to care for.

We would like to thank the authors for their willingness to contribute to this volume and their considerable efforts to meet the editorial demands. We also thank Deborah Reece and Colleagues from John

Wiley & Sons Ltd., Chichester, UK, for their initiative, efficiency and support.

Frank Snoek and Chas Skinner

References

Anderson BJ, Rubin RR (eds). *Practical Psychology for Diabetes Clinicians. How to Deal with the Key Behavioral Issues Faced by Patients and Health Care Teams*. Alexandria: American Diabetes Association, 1996.
Bradley C (ed.). *Handbook of Psychology and Diabetes*. Chur, Switzerland: Harwood, 1994.

Foreword to the Second Edition

It is difficult to conceive of a disease more likely to cause psychological problems than diabetes. Both Type 1 and Type 2 diabetes are lifelong incurable conditions with a strong heritable element, giving plenty of time for the development of guilt and recrimination within a family. Children who develop Type 1 diabetes are 'punished' by a series of injections and blood tests, a diet which forces them to eat when they don't want to and the prohibition of chocolate and ice cream, previously used to reward them for being 'good'. Type 2 diabetes develops largely because individuals make the 'wrong' lifestyle choices during their lives. Furthermore, the consequences of failing to follow an arduous and often painful treatment of limited effectiveness are a series of progressive, devastating complications which can result in blindness, amputation and premature death from cardiovascular disease.

Yet for many years, health care professionals failed to understand the psychological needs of those with diabetes under their care. Treatment was based on an acute health care model with patients waiting, often for hours in crowded waiting rooms, to see a doctor for just a few minutes (in some clinics they were not even permitted to sit down during a consultation!), who would adjust the insulin or medication and then send them on their way for another few months.

Perhaps the best example of this lack of insight was the debate which raged around 'brittle diabetes' in the early 1980s. Young people with Type 1 diabetes, usually women, appeared to become unresponsive to subcutaneous insulin treatment leading to appalling metabolic control and repeated admissions, with often severe uncontrolled diabetes for which there seemed to be no obvious cause. To many, it was unthinkable that those affected could be so self-destructive; that they would deliberately omit insulin and put their lives in jeopardy by inducing severe diabetic ketoacidosis. Many researchers spent much money searching for the metabolic defect which explained why intravenous insulin was more effective than insulin delivered subcutaneously. Of course, we now know that almost all cases of repeated admission with uncontrolled diabetes are indeed due to non-cooperation and that such behaviour, particularly during difficult periods such as adolescence, is common. We also realize that to help those with diabetes manage their condition more successfully, as diabetes health care professionals we need to understand human behaviour much more clearly and that means working with experts in that field.

It is difficult to overstate the progress in diabetes care over the last 20 years. We now understand how complex diabetes care is and how important psychological factors are, in determining the success of treatment. We are aware that if individuals with diabetes are to have any chance of managing their disease successfully, they need to have skills as well as knowledge and support from an expert multi-disciplinary team. The progress that has been made is exemplified by this book, edited by two psychologists with wide experience and expertise in the psychological needs of those with diabetes. The appearance of a second edition with chapters ranging from childhood to old age emphasizes the importance of psychological support for diabetes health care professionals when managing patients from the cradle to the grave.

Some of us are lucky to have a clinical psychologist working within our multi-disciplinary teams, facilitating inter-professional working as well as providing a clinical service. However, most units are not this fortunate and have to rely on the occasional input from psychologists or liaison psychiatrists, few of whom have any specialist knowledge or experience of working with individuals with diabetes. Those in this situation will find the distilled wisdom in this book particularly useful in guiding them through a wide variety of problems. It will help them to manage difficult cases and explain the modern approach to self management and education. However, the knowledge encapsulated in theses pages will prove invaluable to anyone who is privileged to provide a professional service to people with diabetes.

Simon Heller
University of Sheffield

Preface to the Second Edition

The appreciation of psychological issues related to the prevention and management of diabetes mellitus has gained increasing attention in recent decades, from both health psychologists and diabetologists. Diabetes is a complex medical condition, largely self-managed by the patient. It is now well recognized that 'the best of both worlds' is needed to address adequately the needs of people living with diabetes. A bio-psychosocial care model is warranted, incorporating the medical, social and psychological dimensions of this highly prevalent chronic condition. A cure for diabetes seems still a long way ahead, but the acute and long-term consequences of the disease can be significantly influenced by competent self-management, medical treatment and psychosocial support. Not surprisingly, we are witnessing a rapid increase in publications on psychosocial research in the field of diabetes. Epidemiological and clinical studies in youths and adults with diabetes bring forward new understandings of behavioural issues, critical for optimizing diabetes management. Modern medical technology alone can not solve the "diabetes problem". Education and psychosocial care, empowering patients in their efforts to self-manage their diabetes and address psychological barriers, are key to achieve satisfactory medical and psychosocial outcomes.

State-of-the-art diabetes care builds on psychological and behavioural principles, not for only those patients with psychological disorders, but for all persons living and coping with diabetes. This handbook aims to be a reference and source of inspiration with respect to psychology in diabetes care for all professionals in the field.

Since the first edition of *Psychology in Diabetes Care* saw the light, in 2000, new developments have taken place in the psychosocial diabetes arena. We are seeing more and more well-designed psychological intervention studies in diabetes. These are, by definition, complex and can be conducted only within a collaborative framework, characterized by multidisciplinary teamwork typical for high quality diabetes care. Of note is also the involvement of psychologists in the development of clinical guidelines for diabetes care at the national and the international level, underscoring the appreciation of psychosocial issues in diabetes management by all stakeholders, i.e. diabetes health care providers, patient associations and professional organisations. The next challenge will be to see these guidelines being implemented in real life. There is still much work to be done, but it is encouraging to see sophisticated psychological intervention studies in diabetes that help us understand which interventions work best for which patients and why. We sincerely hope this second edition will give you thoughts on how to develop services and research that incorporate effective psychological practice.

Chas Skinner, Frank Snoek
February 2005

1

Diabetes in Children

Barbara J. Anderson and **Julienne Brackett**

1.1 Introduction

The results of the Diabetes Control and Complications Trial[1,2] focused the attention of the medical community on the importance of maintaining blood glucose levels as close to the normal range as possible in order to prevent or delay the devastating complications of diabetes. However, translating this message to families coping with this disease in a child presents many challenges and requires a multi-disciplinary team to care for each family.[3,4] Type 1 (insulin-dependent) diabetes is frequently singled out from many other chronic childhood diseases because its successful treatment demands much self-care and family responsibility for implementing a complex treatment regimen.[5,6] When a child is diagnosed with diabetes, the critical tasks of decision-making concerning the child's daily survival and treatment are transferred from health care professionals to the family. Immediately following diagnosis, the family is responsible for carefully balancing multiple daily insulin injections and food intake with physical activity in order to prevent large fluctuations in blood glucose levels, which can interfere with the child's normal growth and development. Frequent blood glucose monitoring is also required to assess this tenuous balance between insulin, food, and activity.

In the psychosocial literature on paediatric diabetes, it is well documented that this complex daily regimen impacts on every aspect of the child's development and family life.[4,7,8] With respect to psychological development, 'good emotional adjustment' is strongly related to better glycaemic control.[7,9,10] Sufficient studies comparing groups of children with diabetes with non-diabetic comparison samples have been conducted using standardized, objective measures that we can confidently conclude that children with diabetes are not a psychologically 'deviant' group.[9,11,12] However, such global studies have not provided much information

Psychology in Diabetes Care   Edited by Frank J. Snoek and T. Chas Skinner
© 2005 John Wiley & Sons, Ltd.

about what it is about diabetes that affects the developing child and almost every aspect of family life.

Therefore, this chapter will focus on identifying and understanding the specific stresses of living with diabetes that the child and parent must confront at each developmental stage between infancy and the 11th year, and the coping responses that lead to healthy psychological and physical outcomes. Because each developmental stage presents different challenges, we will divide the discussion into (1) diabetes in infancy (0–2 years of age), (2) diabetes in toddlers and preschoolers (2–5 years) and (3) diabetes in the school-age child (6–11 years). For each section, we will briefly review the central milestones of normal psychological development and then examine how the treatment demands of diabetes impact on the developmental tasks of each period. Next, we will discuss how diabetes impacts on the family and vice versa. We will also translate research findings into brief recommendations for health care providers to assist in developing services that best meet the changing psychosocial needs of their paediatric patients with diabetes and their families in each of these developmental periods. The final section of the chapter will review some of the risk factors for poor adjustment and diabetes control that have been identified across the whole of childhood.

1.2   Diabetes in Infancy

Psychological development and the impact of diabetes in infancy

Diabetes diagnosed during infancy has a profound effect on the parent–child relationship. For the first two years of life, the central psychological task is the establishment of a mutually strong and trusting emotional attachment between the infant and the primary caregivers.[13,14] The infant's psychological well-being depends on the predictable presence of an adult who meets the infant's physical needs, provides a stable environment and responds to their social advances.

Because type 1 diabetes is relatively rare in infants and toddlers, and symptoms may vary from those commonly seen, young children with diabetes are often misdiagnosed initially.[15] The child may present with acute vomiting and marked dehydration, which is often attributed to gastroenteritis. The diagnosis of type 1 diabetes in infants is often delayed because it is more difficult for parents to detect classic symptoms of diabetes, such as frequent urination, which would signal the need to seek medical attention. Due to such delays and misdiagnoses at diagnosis, infants and toddlers are more likely than older children to be in diabetic ketoacidosis (DKA) and require hospitalization in an intensive care unit. When hospitalized, infants endure disruptions of expected home routines and are often subjected to invasive medical procedures. Once home, the 'trusted' caregivers are required to give injections and perform painful fingersticks on infants who lack the cognitive ability to understand that the procedures are beneficial.[16] Therefore, the diagnosis of diabetes may threaten the infant's development of a trusting relationship with caregivers. In a qualitative study by Hatton and colleagues,[17] mothers of infants and toddlers with diabetes reported feeling a diminished bond with their children and a loss of the ideal mother–child relationship.

Because young children with diabetes are totally dependent on their parents to manage their disease and to recognize dangerous fluctuations in blood glucose, parents must be constantly vigilant.[18] Due to the stress of the day-to-day management of diabetes, many parents are too exhausted and fearful to leave their child in the care of another.[17,18] In addition, finding 'relief' caregivers who are competent and comfortable caring for a young child with diabetes is often extremely difficult, if not impossible.[3,4,18] Therefore, diabetes may put the infant–parent relationship at risk for overdependence and may restrict the positive separation and reunion experiences that are necessary during infancy. In a descriptive study by Sullivan-Bolyai, it was shown that diabetes might also put mothers at risk for physical and emotional problems, given this constant level of stress and responsibility without easily available support systems. This highlights the importance of helping parents identify support systems to reduce the stresses created by a diagnosis of type 1 diabetes.[18]

Family issues: caring for an infant with diabetes

When a child is diagnosed with IDDM during the first two years of life, the parent(s) or caregiver(s) become the real 'patient'. The grief experienced by parents of infants after diagnosis is often stronger and more emotionally disruptive than when a child is diagnosed at an older age because parents of young infants have more recently celebrated the birth of a 'healthy, perfect' child. In addition, infants are more often critically ill at diagnosis, and the parents may have witnessed their child being cared for in an intensive care unit. This heightens the trauma already experienced by the parent(s), and emphasizes the vulnerability of their child as well as the seriousness of diabetes. After the acute crisis abates, the parents of a very small child are now faced with the reality and implications of the diagnosis. They may find it extremely difficult, both psychologically and physically, to inject insulin into or to take a drop of blood from their infant's tiny body. Parents have described feeling 'riveted to a totally inflexible regimen that ruled their very existence'[17] (p. 572). Parents not only grieve for the loss of a 'healthy' child, but also for the loss of spontaneity, flexibility, and freedom to which they may have been accustomed. In order to ensure that the infant's medical needs are constantly monitored, major lifestyle changes are frequently required.[17] For all of these reasons, the diagnosis of IDDM during infancy is emotionally devastating and extremely stressful to parents. Many parents report that the diagnosis of diabetes increased strain in their marriages and heightened miscommunication between spouses, as well as leading to feelings of depression.[17] However, with time and knowledge, parents in the studies by Hatton *et al.* and Sullivan-Bolyai *et al.* felt greater confidence and found more flexibility in the management regimen, which contributed to adaptation.[17,18] Even as they felt more adapted, the many stresses of diabetes continued to evoke emotional responses.[17]

1.3   Diabetes in Toddlers and Preschoolers

Psychological development and the impact of diabetes: ages 2–5 years

Diabetes during the second to fourth years of life continues to have a profound effect on the parent–child relationship. At this developmental period, the toddler's two central psychological tasks are (1) to separate from the parent or primary caregiver and to establish him/herself as a separate person, by developing a sense of autonomy, with more clearly defined boundaries between the child and the parent, and (2) to develop a sense of mastery over the environment and the confidence that he/she can act upon and produce results in the environment, including the people making up his/her social environment.[13,14]

The restrictions of diabetes management and parental fear stemming from diabetes stress the normal drive of toddlers to explore and master their environments. The toddler's sense of autonomy can be threatened by overprotective caregivers, who may be unable to let the child out of their sight. Out of fear, the parents may scold toddlers for exploring, which can lead to feelings of guilt and shame.[19] The autonomy that a child does develop is often reflected in refusals to cooperate with injections or blood glucose monitoring, as well as in conflicts over food. Toddlers can learn to use food to manipulate their parents, who are afraid of hypoglycaemia, causing the dinner table to become a battleground. Parents of young children with diabetes in a study by Powers *et al.* reported more behavioral feeding problems and mealtime parenting problems than did parents of healthy control subjects.[20] These problems can lead to poor nutritional intake as well as increasing the already high level of parental stress. Although the diabetes management tasks must be carried out, parents can help foster the developing sense of autonomy by allowing the toddler to choose between two injection sites or fingers for blood samples.[19]

As the child reaches the preschool years, the central developmental task becomes the use of the newly established sense of autonomy to investigate the world outside the home. The child is involved in gaining a sense of gender identity, in developing new cognitive abilities that allow more cause–effect thinking, and in separating successfully from parents for the first 'school' experience.[13,14] At this developmental stage, the child must learn to adapt to the expectations of other adults, to trust these adults to provide for his or her needs, and to begin to form relationships with peers and adults outside the family. The child takes increasing initiative to explore and master new skills in environments outside the home.

For preschool-aged children with diabetes, meeting their peers may lead to the first awareness that they are 'different' from other children, in terms of eating, checking blood glucose levels, or wearing medical identification jewellery. As children with diabetes recognize that they are somehow different from others, it is common for them to believe that diabetes is a form of punishment. During this developmental stage, the child is developing his or her own explanations and perceptions of the world. Because diabetes plays a large role in the child's life, the child uses developing, but limited, ideas of causality to reason that diabetes and its painful treatment are the result of his or her bad behaviour.[16]

Given the toddler's and preschooler's normal developmental tasks of establishing their independence from the parent, diabetes only fuels the parent–child conflicts so typical of these stages. Unfortunately, in previous research studies, infants and toddlers with diabetes have been grouped with children under 6 years of age, and studied as a 'preschool sample', yielding little data on these stages specifically. One empirical research study by Wysocki and colleagues[12] has studied the psychological adjustment of very young children from the mothers' perspective, with a sample of 20 children, 2–6 years of age, with a mean age of approximately 4 years. The authors indicated that mothers reported that their children showed significantly more 'internalizing' behaviour problems on the standardized Child Behavior Checklist (CBCL),[21] such as symptoms of depression, anxiety, sleep problems, somatic complaints or withdrawal. However, the authors emphasize that mothers did not rate their toddler and preschool children with diabetes in the clinically deviant range as measured on this standardized instrument.[12] In contrast to the findings of Wysocki et al., Northam and colleagues[22] found no significant deviations from normative scores on any scale of the CBCL at diagnosis or 1 year later in a sample of 18 children under 4 years of age. In both studies, there were no assessments made of the children's behaviour independent of maternal report in either study. This is important to note in light of the other major finding by Wysocki and colleagues, that mothers of very young children with diabetes reported more overall stress in their families when contrasted with a non-diabetic standardization sample, citing the child with diabetes as the source of that stress.[12] Powers et al. also found higher stress levels in parents of children with diabetes compared with parents of non-diabetic children.[20] Despite the cautious interpretation these authors gave to their findings, it is possible that a non-diabetic standardization sample is an inappropriate comparison group. Both Eiser[23] and Garrison and McQuiston[24] have suggested that these types of behavioral change in the young child and changes in parental expectations are to be expected when *any* chronic illness is present in the child. Therefore, it is important not to conclude from these findings that it is diabetes per se that causes the behavioral adjustment problems or that all mothers of preschoolers with diabetes see their families as severely stressed. Clearly, more research into the psychological adjustment of very young children with diabetes and their families is needed. In addition, independent assessments of adjustment need to be used, rather than relying solely on parental report, which can be affected by feelings of guilt or pity.[22]

Family issues: parenting toddlers and preschoolers with diabetes

As is true for infants with diabetes, when a toddler or preschooler has diabetes, the parent(s) or caregiver(s) is the real 'patient'.[3] Parents continue to be responsible for making complex, clinical decisions, and for vigilantly monitoring the child for symptoms of hypoglycaemia. As the child experiences growth spurts, parents often struggle to maintain the child's blood sugar within a safe and acceptable range: a struggle made more difficult by the child's inability to understand the importance of the regimen, and the toddler's inability to verbalize symptoms of high or low blood glucose. Compared to findings from a sample of older children and adolescents with diabetes, mothers of very young children report more concerns about identifying hypoglycaemia, and perceive greater family disruption from diabetes.[12,25] Adding to the parents' stress, toddlers and preschoolers, who are getting physically stronger, may actively resist and refuse insulin injections, blood monitoring, or needed meals and snacks. Restraining the squirming child at injection time or forcing the child to eat may be necessary but extremely stressful for parents who begin to feel that they are 'feeding the insulin, not the child'[17] (p. 573). The children can now also verbalize their fear and anger about invasive procedures, which can devastate parents as these emotions are usually directed at them.[17]

Once children begin to test their autonomy, it is important for parents to set limits and discipline their children appropriately. Temper tantrums are common among young children, hence the phrase 'terrible twos', but they may also signal hypoglycaemia in children with diabetes. Many parents report difficulty distinguishing diabetes-related mood swings from normal toddler behaviour.[17] Once hypoglycaemia has been ruled out through blood glucose monitoring, parents need to set limits and have clear expectations for the child as they would for a child without diabetes. Unfortunately, feelings of guilt or pity about the child's disease may interfere with such limit-setting.[19,26]

Hatton and colleagues report that anticipation of a child entering preschool and being entrusted to another's care can cause much anxiety and concern for parents.[17] Overprotectiveness and pity for a child suffering from separation anxiety can tempt parents to cancel or delay plans for preschool education or daycare, but doing so can thwart the child's growing sense of independence and development of social skills.[19]

1.4 Treatment Issues for Children Under 6 Years of Age

Once diagnosed, the basic goals of diabetes therapy for children under the age of 6 years are similar to those recommended to all children and adolescents and include the avoidance of high and low blood glucose levels and the maintenance of normal growth and development. However, due to the continued development of the central nervous system, young children are particularly vulnerable to the debilitating consequences of recurrent hypoglycaemia.

There is a growing body of evidence supporting the negative consequences, mild, cognitive deficits, resulting from overly aggressive attempts to normalize metabolism in young children. Ack et al.[27] reported modest cognitive deficits in patients with a younger age of onset of type 1 diabetes. Others also reported brain damage as a result of severe hypoglycaemia, particularly in young children.[28,29] A series of studies by Ryan et al.,[30–32] using a battery of neurobehavioural tests, identified significant differences between youth with diabetes compared with control subjects on measures of verbal intelligence, visual–motor coordination, and critical flicker threshold. Additionally, children diagnosed with diabetes under 5 years of age manifested significant cognitive deficits when evaluated during the adolescent years, probably resulting from symptomatic or asymptomatic hypogly-caemia occurring earlier in life before final maturation of the central nervous system. In another study by Rovet et al.,[33] children diagnosed under 4 years of age scored lower than other children with diabetes diagnosed later in childhood and lower than non-diabetic sibling controls on tests of visual–spatial orientation but not on verbal ability. Hypoglycaemic seizures were found to occur with greater frequency in the group of children diagnosed under 4 years of age compared with those diagnosed at older ages, suggesting that severe hypoglycaemia may impair later cognitive functioning.[33]

Golden and colleagues[34] collected longitudinal data on the frequency of hypo-glycaemia from the time of diagnosis in a sample of 23 children with diabetes onset prior to the age of 5 years. Correlating this data with subscale scores on the Stanford–Binet Intelligence Scale yielded no significant findings between fre-quency of severe hypoglycaemia and any of the subscales. Importantly, it was the frequency of asymptomatic and mildly symptomatic hypoglycaemia that was significantly correlated with lower scores on the abstract/visual reasoning scale, indicating that even mild or asymptomatic episodes of hypoglycaemia can have a negative cumulative effect on cognitive functioning.

In the previously described studies, no measurements of neurocognitive func-tioning were made near the time of diagnosis to rule out the possibility that the metabolic decompensation of diabetes onset affected such functioning. Two studies have followed children with diabetes prospectively from diagnosis using neuropsychological assessments. The preliminary findings of Rovet and collea-gues[35] indicated no evidence of neurocognitive impairment in these children at diagnosis or one year later, but the authors reported that they may not have followed subjects long enough to observe any impairment. Northam and collea-gues[36] compared the performance of children with type 1 diabetes on standardized measures of general intelligence, attention, speed of processing, memory, learning, and executive skills with the performance of control subjects. At 3 months post-diagnosis there were no differences between groups, but at 2 years post-diagnosis children with diabetes demonstrated smaller gains, particularly in the areas of information processing speed, acquisition of new knowledge, and conceptual reasoning skills. The subset of the diabetes sample that performed the worst were those children with early onset of diabetes, which further suggests an early onset effect.[36]

In light of these findings, suggesting that even asymptomatic hypoglycaemia in young children with developing nervous systems can be deleterious, prevention of severe and recurrent hypoglycaemia is of paramount importance.[27–40] In addition, infants and toddlers are unable to verbalize when they are suffering from hypoglycaemia, which can lead to delayed treatment, unconsiousness, and/or seizures. A retrospective review of patients less than 9 years of age at Mayo clinic found that 45–55 per cent of children under 5 years of age had experienced severe hypoglycaemic reactions compared with 13 per cent of children between 5 and 9 years of age.[41] The current trend of intensive insulin therapy as advocated by the Diabetes Control and Complications Trial[1,2] for persons over 13 years of age must be implemented very cautiously in these vulnerable young patients.[14,37–41] Therefore, age-specific blood glucose target ranges with the provision for wide glycaemic excursions should be the rule rather than the exception.

Achieving optimal glycaemic control in this age range is further complicated by the finicky eating habits, erratic physical activity, and rapid growth of young children. Treatment goals must therefore be individualized to provide safe and effective medical treatment, yet also permit the young child to master the normal developmental tasks of childhood. For example, the toddler who is a picky, pokey eater may be best suited to rapid-acting insulin analogue injections after meals rather than prior to the meals in order to avoid frantic parents who are unable to 'force' their child to eat. Such insulin administration techniques may reduce the mealtime stresses experienced by many families of toddlers with diabetes.

In recent years, continuous subcutaneous insulin infusion therapy, or 'pump' therapy, has increasingly been used in young children. Several studies have shown that insulin pump therapy is a safe alternative to multiple daily insulin injections and may be associated with improved quality of life for families coping with diabetes.[42–46] One of the most significant findings for parents of young children with diabetes is the reduced rates of severe hypoglycaemic reactions associated with insulin pump therapy.[44–48] In a randomized, controlled study of pump therapy in preschoolers by DiMeglio et al. did not find clinically significant differences in glycaemic control in preschool patients on pump therapy versus intensive multiple daily injections or differential frequency of several hypoglycaemias in patients. However 95 per cent of families randomized to pump therapy during the study continued such therapy after the study period.[43] Pump therapy also allows greater convenience and lifestyle flexibility, such as meal timing, as parents can adjust the timing of insulin bolus delivery in the same manner as using rapid acting analogues. Interestingly, Litton *et al.* found that the frequency of parental contact with their health care providers decreased by 80 per cent after starting pump therapy, which they interpreted as a reflection of increased parental confidence with their diabetes management skills.[44]

Based on these studies, it appears that continuous subcutaneous insulin infusion therapy is an effective treatment alternative for young children. However, long-term outcome studies of children started on pump therapy as infants or toddlers are needed, especially in light of the finding of increased episodes of mild hypoglycaemia by DiMeglio *et al.*[43] As with all management issues, the decision to start pump therapy must be individualized to each family's lifestyle and abilities. Pump therapy can be more expensive than injections and requires more training, which may preclude its use in some families.

If multiple daily injections are used, glargine, a recently introduced long-acting insulin analogue with no appreciable peak action, has been shown to significantly reduce hypoglycaemia, especially nocturnal hypoglycaemia, in children.[49,50] By decreasing hypoglycaemic events, which precipitate so much stress for families with a young child with diabetes, it is hoped that these new management tools can continue to improve the quality of life for these families.

Psychosocial recommendations to health care providers

It is essential that health care providers who work in paediatric diabetes appreciate and address the many stresses and demands confronting parents of infants, toddlers and preschoolers with diabetes by promoting the development of clinical services, childcare referral sources, educational materials and support groups for families living with diabetes at these earliest developmental periods. Parents have reported a need for understanding from and collaboration with a health care team.[17,25] Managing diabetes in young children requires an integrated multi-disciplinary team approach in order to adequately address the complex physiological and psychosocial needs of the children and their families.[3] Support groups and educational materials targeted towards families of very young children can also help parents feel less alone and can normalize feelings of guilt, anxiety and fear.[3] The health care team must create a supportive environment by providing 24-hour on call coverage to help parents cope with unexpected problems, especially as they adjust to life with diabetes outside the hospital.[3,7] Reassurance and non-judgmental support for all members of the family is of great value given the emotional challenges of adapting to post-diagnosis life.[17,18]

1.5   Diabetes in School-aged Children

Psychosocial development and diabetes in the school-aged child

The primary developmental tasks of the child during the elementary school years include making a smooth adjustment from the home to the school setting; forming close friendships with children of the same sex; obtaining approval from this peer group; developing new intellectual, athletic and artistic skills and forming a positive sense of self. [13,14]

Psychological development in school-aged children is assessed primarily with respect to the child's sense of self-esteem and the development of peer relationships. In a careful review of the early empirical psychosocial literature on children with diabetes, Johnson concluded that 'most youngsters with diabetes do not have psychological problems, but among those who do, peer relationship difficulties are quite common. Among all of the personality traits assessed, the evidence for peer or social relationship problems seems the strongest' (p. 101).[9]

Studies of self-esteem in school-aged children with diabetes have consistently linked low self-esteem and poor social–emotional adjustment to poorly controlled diabetes.[9,10] Herskowitz-Dumont and colleagues[51] found a significant association between recurrent diabetic ketoacidosis (DKA) over 8 years post-diagnosis and higher ratings of behaviour problems and lower levels of social competence, as measured by psychological testing in the first year after diagnosis. Similarly, Liss et al.[52] found that children who had been hospitalized with DKA in the preceding 12 months reported lower levels of self-esteem and social competence than children who had no episodes of DKA in the same period. In addition, a significantly larger proportion of the DKA group met the diagnostic criteria for at least one psychiatric disorder (88 versus 28 per cent).

Because the development of peer relationships is an important aspect of the school-age years, it is crucial to examine how diabetes interferes with social development. Several older interview studies have shed light on this topic. Bregani et al.[53] emphasized that during this developmental period children with diabetes often begin to feel a heightened sense of frustration and of social stigma from their dietary restrictions. The authors pointed out that the child's emerging self-awareness and ability to reflect on his/her diabetes and to compare him/herself with peers made the child very vulnerable to feelings of inadequacy. Similarly, Zuppinger et al.[54], in interviews with 23 children with diabetes at this age, found that half of the sample identified teasing from peers and difficulty in accommodating meal schedules to school activities as the major difficulties in following the diabetic diet. Leaverton[55] also suggested that the most common resentment of the child with diabetes in the elementary school years is following a planned diet, because it gives an obvious sign to peers that the child is different. In addition to food restrictions and regularity of meal timing, the need for frequent blood glucose monitoring and insulin injections can emphasize differences and make peer acceptance more difficult.[16]

Kovacs and colleagues[56] found in a longitudinal study of school-aged children newly diagnosed with diabetes that 25 per cent of their sample of school-aged children reported being teased by peers about their diabetes. When asked about the most difficult aspects of diabetes, insulin injections and dietary issues were most commonly cited. Despite the difficult regimen and challenges to peer acceptance, children's self-ratings indicated good self-esteem and few signs of emotional distress in the first year of life with diabetes. Children in this study also reported showing their diabetes supplies to their friends and demonstrated glucose testing, which suggested that the children were actively trying to integrate diabetes into their lives.

School issues

Because the school environment presents many opportunities for building self-esteem and developing socialization skills, it is important for the school-aged child with diabetes to participate fully in all activities with as few restrictions as possible in order to facilitate a normal school experience. Children need to understand that, although they have diabetes, they are not 'sick' or 'abnormal'.[16] Participation in school activities helps to minimize the child's sense of being different from peers. Some modifications in a typical school day may need to be made to accommodate diabetes safely, such as the scheduling of lunch and gym classes to prevent hypoglycaemia, but restricting the child from gym classes or school outings only emphasizes differences and may foster a sense of inferiority.[57]

Children with diabetes should also be encouraged to participate in as many extracurricular activities and sports as they choose and as scheduling permits. For all children, such activities can boost self-esteem and feelings of competence. This effect may be particularly important for children with chronic diseases, such as diabetes.[58]

Participation in school is disrupted if the child has unusually high or low blood sugars or if the child uses diabetes to avoid particular classes.[58] In addition, poorly controlled diabetes can lead to frequent or prolonged absences. Such events may result in educational setbacks and interfere with peer relationships, which may contribute to lower self-esteem.[16] Minimizing the occurrence of hypoglycaemia during the school day is crucial in light of findings by Puczynski and colleagues,[59] which indicated that memory and concentration may continue to be impaired even after the physical symptoms of hypoglycaemia have subsided. These findings have important implications for classroom functioning because many students return to their studies after recovering from the physical symptoms when they may not be able to function on a cognitive level as usual. Unfortunately, this study did not determine the length of time cognitive abilities remained impaired, but it did suggest that teachers should consider whether an episode of hypoglycaemia might have affected a student's performance.

Parents and educators need to be aware that neuropsychological studies have consistently reported 'subtle deficits' in verbal intelligence and specific neuropsychological functions such as attention, memory and executive functions in a high-risk subgroup of school-aged children with type 1 diabetes.[60–63] Children who were diagnosed under 4 years of age or who had a history of severe hypoglycaemic seizures are reported to be at risk for these cognitive deficits.[60–63] While these cognitive changes are consistently described as 'subtle', investigations have not been conducted of the practical implications of these cognitive changes with respect to the child's academic or social functioning. One recent study demonstrated that memory functioning was *not* related to the school-aged child's diabetes self-care behaviours, while memory functioning was related to the self-care behaviour of adolescents who were responsible for more of their own diabetes management tasks.[64]

In order for children with diabetes to have as normal a school experience as possible while maintaining optimal diabetes control, it is necessary for parents and health care providers to provide information and guidance to school personnel to outline expectations for the child's care during the school day. It is important for both educators and parents to know that current guidelines for the care of children with type 1 diabetes allow for much more flexibility in meals and snacks than was recommended in the past.[65] Teachers need to be informed of parental preferences relating to what the child is permitted to eat during school hours and whether substitute foods will be provided from home. School personnel must also be informed about the treatment of out-of-range blood glucose levels, the need for snacks during physical activity and the frequency of blood glucose monitoring and insulin administration if such procedures are deemed necessary during school hours. It is essential that families meet with teachers and school nurses before the start of school to provide such information and guidelines and to facilitate co-operation between the school and the family. By communicating with the school regularly throughout the year, families can prevent conflicts, clarify expectations and feel more confident that their child is safe at school.[58]

Family issues

Because studies suggest that participation with peers, positive self-image and regimen flexibility (especially nutritional flexibility) are critical and interrelated goals for the school-aged child with diabetes, parents should avoid unrealistic demands for adherence to a meal, insulin, or monitoring schedule that restricts the elementary-school child from active participation in age-appropriate school and peer activities. The new, revised guidelines for the care of children with type 1 diabetes which permit more liberal carbohydrate intake[66] and more flexibility in timing of meals and snacks[65] may help to reduce the threats to self-esteem and the social stigmatism experienced by these school-aged children with type 1 diabetes in past decades.

1.6 Family Factors Related to Glycaemic Control and Adherence

Due to the relatively small number of children under the age of 6 with diabetes, there have been few, if any, studies on how family environment variables relate to glycaemic control and adherence. For school-aged children, this area has received more attention. Waller and colleagues conducted one of the first empirical studies of families with children with diabetes under the age of 12 years.[67] These authors concluded that for school-aged patients more diabetes-related family guidance and control were linked to better metabolic outcomes, and that diabetes-related parental warmth and caring were important for optimal outcomes. Liss *et al.* had similar findings in her study of children hospitalized with DKA, who also reported lower levels of diabetes-related warmth and caring.[52]

Non-diabetes-specific family factors, such as conflict, stress and family cohesion, have also been linked to glycaemic control and adherence.[68–74] Viner and colleagues[74] found that high levels of family stress were correlated with poorer glycaemic control in children under 12 years of age. In addition, the authors found that social support buffered the impact of general family stress on the children's glycaemic control. The authors emphasized that the relationship between family stress and glycaemic control is '…bi-directional, with poor diabetic control producing family stress, as well as family stress inducing poor control in the child' (p. 420).[74]

In contrast, other investigations have not found relationships between general family factors and metabolic control or treatment adherence in school-aged children.[75–77] Various methodological and sampling issues have been used to explain these different findings with respect to the link between family stress and metabolic outcomes in school-aged children. Kovacs *et al.*,[77] in a longitudinal study of school-aged children newly diagnosed with diabetes, found no relationship between metabolic control and two general measures of family life—parental perceptions of the quality of family life and the quality of the marriage. These authors speculate that 'metabolic control of children may be affected by aspects of family functioning that are too subtle to have been captured by the measures of general functioning used in this study' (p. 413).[77] Moreover, Kovacs and her colleagues also suggest that a link between metabolic control and family factors in school-aged children may be shown by studying other variables that 'mediate the relationship of family life to metabolic control' (p. 413),[77] variables such as family behaviour with respect to regimen tasks. These authors also reported that for a small subset (approximately seven per cent) of their research families poorer ratings of the family environment at diagnosis were related to subsequent poor metabolic control.[57]

A second longitudinal study of school-aged children with newly diagnosed diabetes by Jacobson, Hauser and colleagues[69,78] revealed that the child's perception of family conflict as measured by a general family measure given at diagnosis was the strongest predictor of poor adherence to insulin administration, meal planning, exercise and blood glucose monitoring tasks over a four-year follow-up period.[69] The relationship between family factors and metabolic control was not examined in this report.

The connection between conflict, adherence and glycaemic control was also examined by Miller-Johnson *et al.*[71] In this study, parent–child conflict was a significant correlate of both adherence and glycaemic control. In multivariate analyses, the relationship between conflict and glycaemic control was non-significant when adherence was entered into the model. These results indicate that conflict may interfere with glycaemic control by disrupting treatment adherence. Similarly, in a recent study of parenting styles, regimen adherence and glycaemic control in 4-to-10-year-olds with type 1 diabetes and their parents, 'authoritative parenting' characterized by parental support and affection was related to better regimen adherence and more optimal glycaemic control. The authors suggest that greater parental warmth may improve adherence by reducing family conflict, increasing family cohesion or both.[79] 'Authoritative parenting', which describes a parenting style in which conflict is minimized as parents set consistent, realistic limits on children's behaviour while displaying warmth and sensitivity to their child's needs and feelings, has been linked to improved behavioural outcomes in the general child development research literature as well as in these empirical studies in school-aged children with type 1 diabetes.[80] Finally, family environments that are more structured and rule governed are associated with better glycaemic control in school-aged children with type 1 diabetes, but not in adolescents.[81]

1.7 Family Involvement in the Diabetes Management of a School-Aged Child

One area of importance for families and health care providers concerns issues of transferring diabetes care responsibilities from the parent to the child.[82] The expanding skills and increased cognitive abilities of the elementary school child make it seem reasonable to transfer more and more daily diabetes care responsibilities. However, there is a growing consensus among recent empirical studies that children and adolescents given greater responsibility for their diabetes management make more mistakes in their self-care, are less adherent and are in poorer metabolic control than those whose parents are more involved.[83–88] Studies using diabetes-specific instruments have consistently found that older children assuming greater responsibility for the tasks of the treatment regimen are in poorer metabolic control than those who assumed less responsibility.[85,89–91]

In her important review of the empirical literature on family responsibility sharing in diabetes, Follansbee[92] concluded 'Cumulatively, these studies yield important information about the role of parent–child interaction in influencing youngsters' assumption of diabetes management. It seems that interdependence, rather than independence, is a worthwhile goal' (p. 350).[92]

From these studies, it has become increasingly clear that parental involvement in diabetes management is required throughout the school-age developmental period. Each family needs to negotiate its own acceptable pattern of parent–child teamwork, based on factors such as child temperament and parent availability. By identifying *shared responsibility* rather than *child independence* as the expectation for school-age children with diabetes, the health care team can help make parent involvement seem less inappropriate to the child or family. It is imperative that the family hears a clear message that diabetes management tasks must be protected from the child's normal drive to achieve independent mastery.

1.8   Treatment Issues for School-aged Children

The goals of diabetes therapy for school-aged children are to avoid severe metabolic decompensation (diabetic ketoacidosis), maintain normal height and weight, minimize the debilitating symptoms of either severely high or low blood glucose levels, establish and maintain a healthy psychosocial environment for the child and family and maintain the involvement of family members in carrying out daily injections and blood sugar monitoring. At this age, children may be more able developmentally and intellectually to recognize and appropriately treat hypoglycaemia. Thus, as the child exits the preschool period, the diabetes team can now work together with the family towards improved glycaemic control, with lower target blood glucose values. A recent study using the well-validated Child Health Questionnaire (CHQ) reported that *psychosocial indices* of well-being were better for children 5–11 years of age with type 1 diabetes who were in good control (HbAlc less than 8.8 per cent), while *physical indices* of well-being did not differ between youngsters in good control and those in poor control (HbAlc greater than 8.8 per cent).[93] Data from Sweden and the US document that there is a limit to the extent to which lowering HbAlc may improve psychosocial and physical quality of life in children with diabetes, with severe episodes of hypoglycaemia associated with the lowest health-related quality of life in children and their parents.[94–96] Thus, while attempting to improve glycaemic control, it is also important for the health care providers to develop treatment regimens that are minimally interruptive to the child's school day and that balance within the child's life the risks of hypoglycaemia with the benefits of optimal control.

Overall, the diabetes treatment team must try to teach problem-solving skills to the parent(s) and child to allow flexibility in the diabetes treatment plan. Similar to the preschool period, diabetes management therapy for the school-aged child is often reactive rather than predictive. During the elementary school years the family continues to be the 'patient'. Parents are an important part of every medical office visit, and parents maintain telephone communication for follow-up at home. At the same office visit, the child and family may see more than one member of the diabetes care team. Because the child grows rapidly during this developmental period, frequent adjustments are needed in the meal plan. Therefore, school-aged children should see the nutritionist at least once each year. The mental health specialist on the team can be especially important in the prevention and negotiation of conflicts over diabetes care issues between the parents and others (such as school personnel) while the child is away from home. To ensure a safe school environment for the child, members of the health care team must be willing to help families communicate guidelines and expectations to school personnel. Diabetes information sheets, with the phone number of the team, should be available for families to provide to the schools.

1.9   Disease Course and Risk Factors: Implications for Clinical Practice

The groundwork for understanding stages of the disease course in diabetes has been laid by three major longitudinal investigations that have followed school-aged children recently diagnosed with IDDM over the early years of their disease. Two research teams followed recently diagnosed children and families over their first decade of life with diabetes.[69,78,97–100] The third investigation, by Grey and colleagues,[101] studied a newly diagnosed cohort of children carefully over their first two years of living with diabetes.

The longitudinal study by Kovacs *et al.*[98,99] followed patients from 2–3 weeks after diagnosis for 6 years. At the end of the first year, the initial emotional distress of both parents and children seemed to have resolved.[102,103] However, results from yearly evaluations indicated that as the duration of diabetes increased patients' emotional distress about diabetes management again increased. Children rated the management regimen as more difficult the longer they had diabetes.[98] This result contrasted with the finding that mothers of these children found it easier to cope with type 1 diabetes as duration increased.[99] The finding that the mothers found it easier to cope with diabetes as duration increased 'could reflect that the children had to take increasing responsibility for (their own) diabetes care' (p. 630).[98] Despite finding it easier to cope with diabetes, the level of emotional symptomatology in mothers also increased slightly after the first year. In addition, these longitudinal studies provided much evidence that initial emotional distress in both children and parents predicted later levels of such distress.[98,99] These studies indicate that clinicians may need to closely monitor children and their parents for signs of emotional distress as disease duration increases in order to intervene early, especially if the family was initially unusually distressed.

Kovacs et al.[100] also examined 'non-compliance with medical treatment' and demonstrated that one in two patients will become non-compliant to the point of endangering their health. Non-compliance or non-adherence emerged at an average of 3.5 years post-diagnosis and at an average age of 15 years, indicating that years three and four following the diagnosis of type 1 diabetes as well as the adolescent period may be particularly high-risk times for non-compliance. The authors suggest that the period of time between diagnosis and the onset of adherence problems may reflect a critical period of adaptation to diabetes, and that, because a low recovery rate was found with non-compliance, interventions to prevent its development are needed during the early period of adaptation.

Adherence to the treatment regimen was also a focus of the longitudinal studies of Jacobson, Hauser and colleagues[69,78,97] in which patients were followed from within the first 9 months of diagnosis. Jacobson et al.[78] reported that, within this patient cohort of newly diagnosed children and adolescents, patients who were school aged at diagnosis (<13 years) had better adherence over a four year follow-up period than did patients who were older (>12 years) at diagnosis. Similarly, Jacobson et al.[97] found that initial child reports of self-esteem, social functioning and adjustment predicted subsequent adherence. Data from this longitudinal study revealed that 'patterns of adherence established early in Year 1 are maintained over time' (p. 523),[78] although deterioration in adherence occurred as duration increased. In addition, they found that the strongest predictor of treatment adherence four years after diagnosis was the child-reported level of family conflict near the time of diagnosis.[69]

Data from this prospective study also indicate that, early in the course of the disease, youth with type 1 diabetes establish a pattern of glycaemic level and regularity of medical appointment-keeping.[104] Youth with the best glycaemic control in the first four years of IDDM who also maintained regular medical follow-up had the lowest incidence of retinopathy outcomes 10–12 years after diagnosis. Assessments of family psychosocial variables, such as cohesiveness, conflict and expressiveness, taken near diagnosis, indicated that a more favourable family environment (i.e. more cohesive and less conflicted) was associated with less deterioration in glycaemic control and fewer acute complications of diabetes, such as DKA and severe hypoglycaemia.[51–72] Based on such findings, family environment at the time of diagnosis and early clinic attendance and adherence should be considered when assessing a child's risk for complications and need for services.

Grey et al.[101] studied a cohort of 8–14-year-old children newly diagnosed with diabetes and a non-diabetic, peer comparison group. The researchers reported that children's adjustment problems at diagnosis disappeared at one year post-diagnosis but reappeared at two years post-diagnosis, a pattern similar to that found by

Kovacs et al.[98,99,102,103] Grey et al. argued that, while previous studies have suggested that the period immediately after diagnosis is the most crucial, their data suggest that a second 'critical period' of adjustment occurs in the second year after diagnosis, and that intervention is important during the critical second year of life with diabetes for prevention of psychosocial deterioration.[101]

These longitudinal studies over the course of diabetes in children have revealed three important points for health care providers. First, a period of difficulty in adjusting to diabetes appears to occur at diagnosis and also during the second year. Second, treatment adherence patterns seem to be established in the early years, two to four years post-diagnosis. Third, family functioning and adjustment assessments may be important predictors of later adherence and diabetes control. The results of these studies indicate that interventions should be carried out after diagnosis before poor adherence patterns can be established. The logical point for multidisciplinary family-centred interventions, which will support adherence to the rigorous treatment regimen by children and families, is therefore in the early years post-diagnosis. Similarly, a recent study comparing the adjustment experiences of parents of youngsters with type 1 diabetes with parents of children diagnosed with cancer reported that the timing of interventions is important early in the disease course, as well as later, when the school-aged child confronts new developmental challenges at adolescence.[105]

Several other important risk factors for poor diabetes control have been investigated in cross-sectional studies. Auslander and colleagues[106,107] found that African-American youths are in significantly poorer glycaemic control than Caucasian youths. Lower levels of adherence in African-American youths contributed to this difference, as did a higher prevalence of single-parent homes. However, both family structure and racial group were confounded with family socio-economic status. Single-parent families have been linked to poorer diabetes outcomes in several studies.[106–108] In a study of correlates of illness severity at diagnosis, children from single-parent homes tended to have more severe symptoms of diabetes, such as DKA, than those living in two-parent families, suggesting that the stress of single parenting and insufficient resources or support may prevent some single parents from seeking medical attention earlier in the disease course.[109] In a single-parent household, the entire burden of diabetes management falls on one parent, who may have less time to devote to the family due to the necessity to work. Financial resources are also typically more limited. Therefore, stress levels in such households may be higher than in two-parent homes. As discussed earlier, family stress has been correlated to glycaemic control in several studies.[68–74] Auslander et al.[70] found that levels of family resources were also strongly related to glycaemic control. Furthermore, lower socioeconomic levels have been implicated as a risk factor for poor glycaemic control and recurrent hospitalizations.[106,110] In light of the findings of these studies, it is crucial for health care providers to assess, at diagnosis and on an ongoing basis, the resources (financial, social and emotional) of the family of a child with diabetes.

Although other minority groups need to be studied in relation to diabetes control, it seems reasonable to suggest that children from single-parent, low socio-economic status and/or minority homes be closely followed to assure early intervention if diabetes control deteriorates.

1.10 Conclusions

In the 21st century, it is possible to have a strong, *optimistic* viewpoint about the futures of children with type 1 diabetes. In the context of improvements in treatment technologies[111] and treatment recommendations,[1,2,65] we confront a future in which the acute and the chronic physical complications of type 1 diabetes for children can more readily be prevented. In addition, two decades of behavioural research with children with type 1 diabetes and their families have helped to make it possible to identify some of the 'predictable crises'[112] that occur as the child moves through the stages of normal growth and development and the phases of diabetes, as well as to identify critical family environment variables that support diabetes management and optimal glycaemic control. We have been encouraged by these recent treatment and research advances, and therefore, in this chapter, we have attempted to identify the intersection between research focused on behavioural and family issues in children with diabetes and diabetes treatment, with the goal of illustrating the potential for prevention of certain behavioural and family 'complications' in childhood diabetes. Armed with a more comprehensive, developmental understanding of the impact of diabetes and its treatment on growing children and their parents, diabetes health care teams can work to prevent problems or to intervene before problems overwhelm families, and thereby improve the quality of life for children and families living with diabetes. Above all, health care providers must strive to provide a family-based model of care, recognizing the impact that diabetes has on *all* members of the family.

Within the current era of competition for health care resources, it becomes even more critical to ensure that the prevailing philosophy of 'doing less' does not move us backwards in the diabetes care of children and adolescents. Now, more than ever before, a multidisciplinary team is critical for the appropriate translation of advances such as the DCCT recommendations and for the prevention of problems—such as severe hypoglycaemia in the preschool period or premature responsibility for diabetes management by older children—that have plagued previous cohorts of children and families. Now that we can offer hope for a healthy future to young patients, as health care providers and investigators, we must discover the energy and vision to create feasible health care systems to deliver this improved, more advanced and comprehensive treatment for type 1 diabetes to children and their families.

References

1. Diabetes Control and Complications Trial Research Group. The effect of intensive treatment of diabetes on the development and progression of long-term complications in insulin-dependent diabetes mellitus. *N Engl J Med* 1993; **329**: 977–986.

2. Diabetes Control and Complications Trial Research Group. Effect of intensive diabetes treatment on the development and progression of long-term complications in adolescents with insulin-dependent diabetes mellitus: Diabetes Control and Complications Trial. *J Pediatr* 1994; **125**: 177–188.

3. Kushion W, Salisbury PJ, Seitz KW, Wilson BE. Issues in the care of infants and toddlers with insulin dependent diabetes mellitus. *Diabetes Educ* 1991; **17**: 107–110.

4. Wolfsdorf JI, Anderson BA, Pasquarello C. Treatment of the child with diabetes. In Kahn CR, Weir G (eds), *Joslin's Diabetes Mellitus*, 13th edn. Philadelphia, PA: Lea Febiger, 1994, pp 430–451.

5. Anderson BJ, Auslander WF. Research on diabetes management and the family: a critique. *Diabetes Care* 1980; **3**: 696–702.

6. Curtis JA, Hagerty D. Managing diabetes in childhood and adolescence. *Can Fam Physician* 2002; **48**: 505–509.

7. Silverstein JH, Johnson S. Psychosocial challenge of diabetes and the development of a continuum of care. *Pediatr Ann* 1994; **23**: 300–305.

8. Faulkner MS, Clark FS. Quality of life for parents of children and adolescents with type 1 diabetes. *Diabetes Educ* 1998; **24**: 721–727.

9. Johnson SB. Psychological factors in juvenile diabetes: a review. *J Behav Med* 1980; **3**: 95–116.

10. Ryden O, Nevander L, Johnsson P, Hansson K, Kronvall P, Sjoblad S, Westbom L. Family therapy in poorly controlled juvenile IDDM: effects on diabetes control, self-evaluation, and behavioral symptoms. *Acta Paediatr* 1994; **83**: 285–291.

11. Jacobson AM, Hauser ST, Wertlieb D, Wolfsdorf JI, Orleans J, Vieyra M. Psychological adjustment of children with recently diagnosed diabetes mellitus. *Diabetes Care* 1986; **9**: 323–329.

12. Wysocki T, Huxtable K, Linscheid TR, Wayne W. Adjustment to diabetes mellitus in pre-schoolers and their mothers. *Diabetes Care* 1989; **12**: 524–529.

13. Erikson EH. *Childhood and Society*. New York: Norton, 1950.

14. Erikson EH. *Identity: Youth and Crisis*. New York: Norton, 1968.

15. Bland GL, Wood VD. Diabetes in infancy: diagnosis and current management. *J Natl Med Assoc* 1991; **83**: 361–365.

16. Pond JS, Peters ML, Pannell DL, Rogers CS. Psychosocial challenges for children with insulin-dependent diabetes mellitus. *Diabetes Educ* 1995; **21**: 297–299.

17. Hatton DL, Canam C, Thorne S, Hughes AM. Parents' perceptions of caring for an infant or toddler with diabetes. *J Adv Nurs* 1995; **22**: 569–577.

18. Sullivan-Bolyai S, Deatrick J, Gruppuso P, Tamborlane W, Grey M. Constant vigilance: mothers' work parenting young children with type 1 diabetes. *J Pediatr Nurs* 2003; **18**: 21–29.

19. Lipman TH, Difazio DA, Meers RA, Thompson RL. A developmental approach to diabetes in children: birth through preschool. *MCN Am J Matern Child Nurs* 1989; **14**: 255–259.

20. Powers SW, Byars KC, Mitchell MJ, Patton SR, Standiford DA, Dolan LM. Parent report of mealtime behavior and parenting stress in young children with type 1 diabetes and in healthy control subjects. *Diabetes Care* 2002; **25**: 313–318.

21. Achenbach TM, Edelbrock CS. *Manual for the Child Behavior Checklist and Revised Child Behavior Profile*. Burlington, VT: University of Vermont Press, 1983.

22. Northam E, Anderson P, Adler R, Werther G, Warne G. Psychosocial and family functioning in children with insulin-dependent diabetes at diagnosis and one year later. *J Pediatr Psychol* 1996; **21**: 699–717.
23. Eiser C. *Chronic Childhood Disease: an Introduction to Psychological Theory and Research*. New York: Cambridge University Press, 1990.
24. Garrison WT, McQuiston S. *Chronic Illness during Childhood and Adolescence*. Newbury Park, CA: Sage, 1989.
25. Banion CR, Miles MS, Carter MC. Problems of mothers in management of children with diabetes. *Diabetes Care* 1983; **6**: 548–551.
26. Yoos L. Chronic childhood illness: developmental issues. *Pediatr Nurs* 1987; **13**: 25–28.
27. Ack M, Miller I, Weil WB. Intelligence of children with diabetes mellitus. *Pediatr* 1961; **28**: 764–770.
28. Bale RN. Brain damage in diabetes mellitus. *Br J Psychiatry* 1973; **122**: 337–391.
29. Holmes CS, Hayford JT, Gonzalez JL, Weydert JA. A survey of cognitive function in different glucose levels in diabetic persons. *Diabetes Care* 1983; **6**: 180–183.
30. Ryan C, Vega A, Longstreet C, Drash A. Neuropsychological changes in adolescents with insulin-independent diabetes. *J Consult Clin Psychol* 1984; **52**: 335–342.
31. Ryan C, Longstreet C, Morrow L. The effects of diabetes mellitus on the school attendance and school achievement of adolescents. *Child: Care, Health, and Development* 1985; **11**: 229–240.
32. Ryan C, Vega A, Drash A. Cognitive deficits in adolescents who developed diabetes early in life. *Pediatr* 1985; **75**: 921–927.
33. Rovet JF, Ehrlich RM, Hoppe M. Intellectual deficits associated with early onset of insulin-dependent diabetes mellitus in children. *Diabetes Care* 1987; **10**: 510–515.
34. Golden MP, Ingersoll GM, Brack CJ, Russell BA, Wright JC, Huberty TJ. Longitudinal relationship of asymptomatic hypoglycaemia to cognitive function in IDDM. *Diabetes Care* 1989; **12**: 89–93.
35. Rovet JF, Ehrlich RM, Czuchta D. Intellectual characteristics of diabetic children at diagnosis and one year later. *J Pediatr Psychol* 1990; **15**: 775–788.
36. Northam EA, Anderson PJ, Werther GA, Warne GL, Adler RG, Andrewes D. Neuropsychological complications of IDDM in children 2 years after disease onset. *Diabetes Care* 1998; **21**: 379–384.
37. Golden MP, Russell BP, Ingersoll GM, Gray DL, Hummer KM. Management of diabetes in children younger than 5 years of age. *Am J Dis Child* 1985; **139**: 448–452.
38. Drash AL. The child, the adolescent, and The Diabetes Control and Complications Trial. *Diabetes Care* 1993; **16**: 1515–1516.
39. Brink SJ, Moltz K. The message of the DCCT for children and adolescents. *Diabetes Spectrum* 1997; **10**: 259–267.
40. Ryan CM, Becker DJ. Hypoglycemia in children with type 1 diabetes mellitus. Risk factors, cognitive function, and management. *Endocrinol Metab Clin North Am* 1999; **28**: 883–900.
41. Lteif AN, Schwenk WF. Type 1 diabetes mellitus in early childhood: glycemic control and associated risk of hypoglycemic reactions. *Mayo Clin Proc* 1999; **74**: 211–216.
42. Shehadeh N, Battelino T, Galatzer A, Naveh T, Hadash A, de Vries L, Phillip M. Insulin pump therapy for 1–6 year old children with type 1 diabetes. *Isr Med Assoc J* 2004; **6**: 284–286.
43. DiMeglio LA, Pottorff TM, Boyd SR, France L, Fineberg N, Eugster EA. A randomized, controlled study of insulin pump therapy in diabetic preschoolers. *J Pediatr* 2004; **145**: 380–384.

44. Litton J, Rice A, Friedman N, Oden J, Lee MM, Freemark M. Insulin pump therapy in toddlers and preschool children with type 1 diabetes mellitus. *J Pediatr* 2002; **141**: 490–495.

45. Saha ME, Huuppone T, Mikael K, Juuti M, Komulainen J. Continuous subcutaneous insulin infusion in the treatment of children and adolescents with type 1 diabetes mellitus. *J Pediatr Endocrinol Metab* 2002; **15**: 1005–1010.

46. Tubiana-Rufi N, de Lonlay P, Bloch J, Czernichow P. Remission of severe hypoglycemic incidents in young diabetic children treated with subcutaneous infusion. *Arch Pediatr* 1996; **3**: 969–976.

47. Bulsara MK, Holman CD, Davis EA, Jones TW. The impact of a decade of changing treatment on rates of severe hypoglycemia in a population-based cohort of children with type 1 diabetes. *Diabetes Care* 2004; **27**: 2293–2298.

48. Weinzimer SA, Doyle EA, Steffen AT, Sikes KA, Tamborlane WV. Rediscovery of insulin pump treatment of childhood type 1 diabetes. *Minerva Med* 2004; **95**: 85–92.

49. Hathout EH, Fujishige L, Geach J, Ischandar M, Mauro S, Mace JW. Effect of therapy with insulin glargine (Lantus) on glycemic control in toddlers, children, and adolescents with diabetes. *Diabetes Technol Ther* 2003; **5**: 801–806.

50. Tan CY, Wilson DM, Buckingham B. Initiation of insulin glargine in children and adolescents with type 1 diabetes. *Pediatr Diabetes* 2004; **5**: 80–86.

51. Herskowitz Dumont R, Jacobson AM, Cole C, Hauser ST, Wolfsdorf JI, Willett JB, Milley JE, Wertlieb D. Psychosocial predictors of acute complications of diabetes in youth. *Diabet Med* 1995; **12**: 612–618.

52. Liss DS, Waller DA, Kennard BD, McIntire D, Capra P, Stephens J. Psychiatric illness and family support in children and adolescents with diabetic ketoacidosis: a controlled study. *J Am Acad Child Adolesc Psychiatry* 1998; **37**: 536–544.

53. Bregani P, Della Porta V, Carbone A *et al*. Attitude of juvenile diabetics and their families towards dietetic regimen. *Pediatr Adoles Endocrinol* 1979; **7**: 159–163.

54. Zuppinger K, Schmid E, Schutz B. Attitude of juvenile diabetics, his family and peers toward a dietetic regimen. *Pediatr Adoles Endocrinol* 1979; **7**: 153–158.

55. Leaverton DR: The child with diabetes mellitus. In Noshpitz JD (ed.), *Basic Handbook of Child Psychiatry*, Vol. I. New York: Basic, 1979, p 452.

56. Kovacs M, Brent D, Steinberg TF, Paulauskas S, Reid J. Children's self-reports of psychologic adjustment and coping strategies during first year of insulin-dependent diabetes mellitus. *Diabetes Care* 1986; **9**: 472–479.

57. Lipman TH, Difazio DA, Meers RA, Thompson RL. A developmental approach to diabetes in children: school-age through adolescence. *MCN Am J Matern Child Nurs* 1989; **14**: 330–332.

58. Balik B, Haig B, Moynihan PM. Diabetes and the school-aged child. *MCN Am J Matern Child Nurs* 1986; **11**: 324–330.

59. Puczynski MS, Puczynski SS, Reich J, Kaspar JC, Emanuele M. Mental efficiency and hypoglycemia. *J Dev Behav Pediatr* 1990; **11**: 170–174.

60. Northam EA, Anderson PJ, Jacobs R, Hughes M, Warne GI, Werther GA. Neuropsychological profiles of children with Type 1 diabetes 6 years after disease onset. *Diabetes Care* 2001; **24**: 1541–1546.

61. Ryan C, Becker D. Hypoglycemia in children with type 1 diabetes mellitus: risk factors, cognitive function, and management. *Endocrinol Metab Clin North Am* 1999; **28**: 883–900.

62. Rovet JF, Ehrlich RM. The effect of hypoglycemic seizures on cognitive function in children with diabetes: a 7-year prospective study. *J Pediatr* 1999; **134**: 503–506.

63. Desrocher M, Rovet JF. Neurocognitive correlates of type 1 diabetes mellitus in childhood. *Neuropsychol Dev Cogn Sect C Child Neuropsychol* 2004; **10**: 36–52.

64. Soutor SA, Chen R, Streisand R, Koplowitz P, Holmes CS. Memory matters: developmental differences in predictors of diabetes care behaviours. *J Pediatr Psychol* 2004; **29**: 493–505.

65. Silverstein J, Klingensmith G, Copeland K, Plotnick L, Kaufman F, Laffel L, Deeb L, Grey M, Anderson B, Holzmeister LA, Clark N. Care of children and adolescents with Type 1 diabetes. *Diabetes Care* 2005; **28**: 186–212.

66. Franz MJ, Horton ES Sr, Bantle JP, Beebe CA, Brunzell JD, Coulston AM, Henry RR, Hoogwerf BJ, Stacpoole PW. Nutrition principles for the management of diabetes and related complications. *Diabetes Care* 1994; **17**: 490–518.

67. Waller D, Chipman JJ, Hardy BW, Hightower MS, North AJ, Williams SB, Babick AJ. Measuring diabetes-specific family support and its relation to metabolic control: a preliminary report. *J Am Acad Child Psychol* 1986; **25**: 415–418.

68. Marteau TM, Bloch S, Baum JD. Family life and diabetic control. *J Child Psychol Psychiat* 1987; **28**: 823–833.

69. Hauser ST, Jacobson AM, Lavori P, Wolfsdorf JI, Herskowitz RD, Milley JE, Bliss R, Gelfand E, Wertlieb D, Stein J. Adherence among children and adolescents with insulin-dependent diabetes mellitus over four-year longitudinal follow-up: II. Immediate and long-term linkages with the family milieu. *J Pediatr Psychol* 1990; **15**: 527–542.

70. Auslander WF, Bubb J, Rogge M, Santiago JV. Family stress and resources: potential areas of intervention in children recently diagnosed with diabetes. *Health Soc Work* 1993; **18**: 101–113.

71. Miller-Johnson S, Emery RE, Marvin RS, Clarke W, Lovinger R, Martin M. Parent–child relationships and the management of diabetes mellitus. *J Consult Clin Psychol* 1994; **62**: 603–610.

72. Jacobson AM, Hauser ST, Lavori P, Willett JB, Cole CF, Wolfsdorf JI, Dumont RH, Wertlieb D. Family environment and glycemic control: a four-year prospective study of children and adolescents with insulin-dependent diabetes mellitus. *Psychosom Med* 1994; **56**: 401–409.

73. Goldston DB, Kovacs M, Obrosky S, Iyengar S. A longitudinal study of life events and metabolic control among youths with insulin-dependent diabetes mellitus. *Health Psychol* 1995; **14**: 409–414.

74. Viner R, McGrath M, Trudinger P. Family stress and metabolic control in diabetes. *Arch Dis Child* 1996; **74**: 418–421.

75. Chase HP, Jackson GG. Stress and sugar control in children with insulin-dependent diabetes mellitus. *J Pediatr* 1981; **98**: 1011–1013.

76. Hauenstein EJ, Marvin RS, Snyder AL, Clarke WL. Stress in parents of children with diabetes mellitus. *Diabetes Care* 1989; **12**: 18–23.

77. Kovacs M, Kass RE, Schnell TM, Goldston D, Marsh J. Family functioning and metabolic control of school-aged children with IDDM. *Diabetes Care* 1989; **12**: 409–414.

78. Jacobson AM, Hauser ST, Lavori P, Wolfsdorf JI, Herskowitz RD, Milley JE, Bliss R, Gelfand E, Wertlieb D, Stein J. Adherence among children and adolescents with insulin-dependent diabetes mellitus over four-year longitudinal follow-up: I. The influence of patient coping and adjustment. *J Pediatr Psychol* 1990; **15**: 511–526.

79. Davis CL, Delamater AM, Shaw KH, LaGreca AM, Eidson MS, Perez-Rodriguez JE. Parenting styles, regimen adherence, and glycemic control in 4–10-year-old children with diabetes. *J. Pediatr Psychol* 2001;**26**: 123–129.

80. Anderson BJ. Family conflict and diabetes management in youth: clinical lessons from child development and diabetes research. *Diabetes Spectrum* 2004; **17**: 22–26.

81. Cohen DM, Lumley MA, Naar-King S, Partridge T, Cakan N. Child behavior problems and family functioning as predictors of adherence and glycemic control in economically

disadvantaged children with Type 1 diabetes: a prospective study. *J Pediatr Psychol* 2004; **29**: 171–184.

82. Parker H, Swift PGF, Botha JL. Early onset diabetes: parents' views. *Diabet Med* 1994; **11**: 593–596.

83. Burns KL, Green P, Chase HP: psychosocial correlates of glycemic control as a function of age in youth with IDDM. *J Adoles Health Care* 1986; **7**: 311–319.

84. Ingersoll GM, Orr DP, Herrold AJ, Golden MP. Cognitive maturity and self-management among adolescents with insulin-dependent diabetes mellitus. *J Pediatr* 1986; **108**: 620–623.

85. Anderson BJ, Auslander WF, Jung KC, Miller JP, Santiago JV. Assessing family sharing of diabetes responsibilities. *J Pediatr Psychol* 1990; **15**: 477–492.

86. Weissberg-Benchell J, Glasgow AM, Tynan WD, Wirtz P, Turek J, Ward J. Adolescent diabetes management and mismanagement. *Diabetes Care* 1995; **18**: 77–82.

87. Wysocki T, Taylor A, Hough BS, Linsheid TR, Yeates KO, Naglieri JA. Deviation for developmentally appropriate self-care autonomy. Association with diabetes outcomes. *Diabetes Care* 1996; **19**: 119–125.

88. Anderson B, Ho J, Brackett J, Finkelstein D, Laffel L. Parental involvement in diabetes management tasks: relationships to blood glucose monitoring adherence and metabolic control in young adolescents with insulin-dependent diabetes mellitus. *J Pediatr* 1997; **130**: 257–265.

89. Allen DA, Tennen H, McGrade BJ, Affleck G, Ratzan S. Parent and child perceptions of the management of juvenile diabetes. *J Pediatr Psychol* 1983; **8**: 129–141.

90. Rubin R, Young-Hyman D, Peyrot M. Parent–child responsibility and conflict in diabetes care. *Diabetes* 1989; **38** (Suppl. 2): 28.

91. LaGreca AM. Children with diabetes and their families: coping and disease management. In Field T, McCabe P, Schneiderman N (eds), *Stress and Coping Across Development*. Hillsdale, NJ: Erlbaum, 1988, pp 139–159.

92. Follansbee DS. Assuming responsibility for diabetes management: What age? What price? *Diabetes Educ* 1989; **15**: 347–352.

93. Wake M, Hesketh K, Cameron FJ. The Child Health Questionnaire in children with diabetes: cross sectional survey of parent and adolescent-reported functional health status. *Diabet Med* 2000; **17**: 700–707.

94. Cameron FJ. The impact of diabetes on health-related quality of life in children and adolescents. *Pediatr Diabetes* 2003; **4**: 132–136.

95. Nordfeldt S, Jonsson D. Short-term effects of severe hypoglycemia in children and adolescents with type 1 diabetes. A cost-of-illness study. *Acta Paediatr* 2001; **90**: 137–142.

96. Marrero DG, Guare JC, Vandagriff JL, Fineberg NS. Fear of hypoglycemia in the parents of children and adolescents with diabetes: maladaptive or healthy response? *Diabetes Educ* 1007; **23**: 281–286.

97. Jacobson AM, Hauser ST, Wolfsdorf JI, Houlihan J, Milley JE, Herskowitz RD, Wertlieb D, Watt BA. Psychologic predictors of compliance in children with recent onset of diabetes mellitus. *J Pediatr* 1987; **110**: 805–811.

98. Kovacs M, Iyengar S, Goldston D, Stewart J, Obrosky DS, Marsh J. Psychological functioning of children with insulin-dependent diabetes mellitus: a longitudinal study. *J Pediatr Psychol* 1990; **15**: 619–632.

99. Kovacs M, Iyengar S, Goldston D. Obrosky DS, Marsh J. Psychological functioning among mothers of children with insulin-dependent diabetes mellitus: a longitudinal study. *J Consult Clin Psychol* 1990; **58**: 189–195.

100. Kovacs M, Goldston D. Obrosky DS, Iyengar S. Prevalence and predictors of pervasive noncompliance with medical treatment among youths with insulin-dependent diabetes mellitus. *J Am Acad Child Adolesc Psychiatry* 1992; **31**: 1112–1119.

101. Grey M, Cameron ME, Lipman TH, Thurber FW. Psychosocial status of children with diabetes in the first 2 years after diagnosis. *Diabetes Care* 1995; **18**: 1330–1336.
102. Kovacs M, Feinberg TL, Paulauskas S, Finkelstein R, Pollock M, Crouse-Novak M. Initial coping responses and psychosocial characteristics of children with insulin-dependent diabetes mellitus. *J Pediatr* 1985; **106**: 827–834.
103. Kovacs M, Finkelstein R, Feinberg TL, Crouse-Novak M, Paulauskas S, Pollock M. Initial psychologic responses of parents to the diagnosis of insulin-dependent diabetes mellitus in their children. *Diabetes Care* 1985; **8**: 568–575.
104. Jacobson AM, Hauser ST, Willet J, Wolfsdorf JI, Herman L. Consequences of irregular vs. continuous medical follow-up in children and adolescents with insulin-dependent diabetes mellitus. *J Pediatr* 1997; **131**: 727–733.
105. Boman KK, Viksten J, Kogner P, Samuelsson U. Serious illness in childhood: the different threats of cancer and diabetes from a parent perspective. *J Pediatr* 2004; **145**: 373–379.
106. Auslander WF, Anderson BJ, Bubb J, Jung KC, Santiago JV. Risk factors to health in diabetic children: a prosective study from diagnosis. *Health Soc Work* 1990; **15**: 133–142.
107. Auslander WF, Thompson S, Dreitzer D, White NH, Santiago JV. Disparity in glycemic control and adherence between African-American and Caucasian youths with diabetes. Family and community contexts. *Diabetes Care* 1997; **20**: 1569–1575.
108. Overstreet S, Goins J, Chen RS, Holmes CS, Greer T, Dunlap WP, Frentz J. Family environment and the interrelation of family structure, child behavior, and metabolic control for children with diabetes. *J Pediatr Psychol* 1995; **20**: 435–447.
109. Charron-Prochownik D, Kovacs M, Obrosky DS, Ho V. Illness characteristics and psychosocial and demographic correlates of illness severity at onset of insulin-dependent diabetes mellitus among school-age children. *J Pediatr Nurs* 1995; **10**: 354–359.
110. Kovacs M, Charron-Prochownik D, Obrosky DS. A longitudinal study of biomedical and psychosocial predictors of multiple hospitalizations among young people with insulin-dependent diabetes mellitus. *Diabet Med* 1995; **12**: 142–148.
111. Wolfsdorf JI, Laffel LMB. Diabetes in childhood: predicting the future. *Pediatr Ann* 1994; **23**: 306–312.
112. Hamburg BA, Inoff GE. Predictable crises of diabetes. *Diabetes Care* 1983; **6**: 409–416.

2

Diabetes in Adolescents

T. Chas Skinner, Helen Murphy and
Michelle V. Huws-Thomas

2.1 Introduction

There is no widely accepted precise definition of what adolescence is, but it is
commonly referred to as the transitional period between childhood and adulthood.
As this is not the place to discuss the social, cultural, historical or political
construction of adolescence, for the purposes of this chapter adolescence is taken
as referring to young people between 12 and 20 years old, thereby mapping fairly
closely the teenage years.

Whatever definition we use, the adolescent years are clearly a period of rapid
change and development. Children progress through the education system to
compete with adults for resources and jobs. This is accompanied by continued
cognitive development, enabling young people to think in increasingly abstract
ways and to become less receptive to authority figures. As they compete for jobs or
higher education places, teenagers are attempting to establish their identity and
lifestyle, and quite early on have to make choices that will affect their long term
career aspirations. Adolescents spend increasing amounts of time away from
home, and their leisure activities become less structured, with ever diminishing
adult supervision or involvement. It is during this period that we learn how to form
and maintain friendships and close intimate relationships with our peers. With
puberty comes the adjustment to a changing body and interest in sexual relationships. The timing of puberty can also have a substantial impact on adolescent
development, with early or late onset of puberty having markedly different effects
on boys' and girls' psycho-social development. With all these changes occurring in
a relatively short period, probably ending with the adoption of lifestyles that will
endure through adulthood, it would seem reasonable to suggest that adolescence

Psychology in Diabetes Care Edited by Frank J. Snoek and T. Chas Skinner
© 2005 John Wiley & Sons, Ltd.

provides us with the opportunity of having a lasting and significant impact on the health and well-being of individuals.

Adolescence is a particularly critical time for young people with diabetes. Whether diagnosed in childhood or adolescence, it is during the adolescent years that the individual learns to take increasing responsibility for the management of their diabetes.[1–3] As they start to integrate their diabetes management tasks into their emerging lifestyles, teenagers directly experience the relationship between their actions and blood glucose tests, if they do any. This will in turn influence their beliefs about diabetes, its treatment and how they will manage it. Therefore these will be formative years in the development of such beliefs, which, once fully integrated and accepted by the young person, may prove difficult to change.

Adolescence is also frequently seen as a time to change and intensify insulin regimens. Whether this is in response to trying to make diabetes management more flexible to fit with the young person's lifestyle, or in an attempt to improve diabetes control, intensifying regimens adds to the demands of diabetes, especially during the adolescent years. The additional pressures to test blood glucose and adjust insulin can mean intensification will result in increasing intrusiveness making the social life of young people even more difficult.

Research consistently demonstrates that during adolescence there is a marked decline in metabolic control.[4–6] Although this decline is partly attributable to the physiological changes occurring at this time,[7,8] the decline in self-care seen during adolescence is of equal if not greater importance.[9–11] This deterioration is particularly marked and of concern in the area of insulin administration. Although self-report data suggested that missed insulin injections were common, the pharmacy record data from the DARTS database demonstrates that about 28 per cent of young adults do not even obtain sufficient insulin to meet their prescribed regimen.[11]

In addition to insufficient insulin resulting in hyperglycaemia, repeated failure to inject insulin can result in diabetic ketoacidosis (DKA). Post-diagnosis recurrent DKA, in the absence of other medical complications, is commonly caused by low levels of insulin administration,[12] with the incidence of recurrent DKA peaking during adolescence.[13]

As if these diabetes burdens were not enough, for many young people especially those diagnosed early in life, their annual review will begin to include screening for the complications of diabetes, adding to their anxieties and emotional burden. It is not surprising then that young people are more likely to drop out of the system and not attend outpatient clinics.[14,15] Furthermore, with the emphasis on monitoring diet and weight, young people, and in particular young females, are at a greater risk of developing disordered eating patterns,[16,17] which may lead to clinical eating disorders.

This brief summary makes it clear that adolescents with diabetes are in the unenviable position of facing the same developmental tasks and demands as other young people, in addition to learning to manage and live with their diabetes. This poses healthcare professionals and parents with numerous challenges as they seek to maintain or improve diabetes control through this transitional phase, without depriving young people of the appropriate age-related experiences to enable development and growth.

This complex array of diabetes and general developmental issues has generated a wealth of literature on the psychological aspects of paediatric chronic illness, and diabetes in particular. However, the literature has seen a marked change in emphasis in recent years, from descriptive research to more intervention based research. In 2000, the National Health Service Health Technology Assessment program published a systematic review of psycho-educational interventions for adolescents.[18] The results of this review data indicated that there were numerous methodological shortcomings in the literature. Only one-half of the interventions were theoretically guided; over one-half of the studies used GHb as an outcome, when it is more appropriate to evaluate the effectiveness of a behavioural intervention in terms of the behaviours it is designed to impact. Follow-up assessments were relatively rare but, to examine maintenance, the long term effectiveness of these interventions needs to be evaluated. Sample sizes were typically small and rarely based on power analyses; effects of ethnicity and socioeconomic status were not examined and cost-effectiveness issues were not addressed.[19] The review identified only a relatively small number of interventions that were reported in sufficient detail to permit the calculation of effect sizes. However, the meta-analysis indicated that,[20] overall, these interventions were effective in the short term and that theoretically based interventions were more effective than atheoretical interventions. Since this review and metanalysis, psycho-educational interventions for adolescents have increased in frequency and both theoretical and empirical rigour. For the purposes of this chapter, the interventions in this review and more recent work can be grouped into three main types, those specifically targeting individuals with persistent poor glycaemic control as evidenced by recurrent ketoacidosis, family-based interventions and those focused on the individual adolescent, rather than the family.

Recurrent ketoacidosis

Diabetic ketoacidosis (DKA) is the single most common cause of mortality in individuals with type 1 diabetes under the age of 40.[21] In addition to the risk of fatality, recurrent DKA has a major impact on the quality of life of both the individuals with diabetes and their families, and microvascular complications may be accelerated. Research shows a number of consistent themes that enable us to identify individuals at potential risk for recurrent DKA, with about 20 per cent of individuals accounting for 80 per cent of hospital admissions for DKA.[22,23]

The incidence is higher in females, peaks in the early teenage years and rarely occurs in anyone diagnosed for less than 2 years. Individuals with earlier age of onset and lower socioeconomic backgrounds seem to be at increased risk, along with individuals who had existing psychopathology before diabetes onset.[22,23] However, there is a distinct lack of evidence for individuals with recurrent DKA to have a subtype of brittle diabetes,[24] and the main cause of DKA is insulin omission. Further long term follow-up data indicates that recurrent DKA is usually not sustained into adulthood.[25,26] This leads to consideration of why some young adolescents persistently omit insulin. There are multiple reasons for this, but the literature seems to point to a relative few main candidates.

There is consistent support for psychosocial risk factors as predictive of recurrent DKA. Individuals from families low in warmth and support, where there are high levels of *unresolved* family conflict and a distinct lack of parental involvement in the adolescent's diabetes care seem to be typical of this population.[26–29] Linked to this is the possibility that the young person may want to escape from the home environment, for reasons of physical, sexual or emotional abuse and or neglect. A recent classic example was a child who omitted her insulin whenever she was due to spend time with her father, her parents being divorced. With some gentle questioning by the care team, she admitted that she did not want to visit with him and the possibility of parental abuse was subsequently confirmed. With subsequent removal of paternal visitation rights the episodes of DKA ceased.

Alternatively, weight manipulation or eating disorders have been shown to be associated with short and long term complications.[30] Although the data on prevalence on eating disorder literature is rather contradictory, with some studies finding elevated rates in people with type 1 diabetes[31–33] whilst other papers do not support this finding,[34–36] a recently published large study with a good control group showed no increase in rates of anorexia or bulimia, but the incidence of eating disorders not otherwise specified (EDNOS) was two to three times as prevalent in young females with type 1 diabetes.[37] Given the perfectionist nature of individuals with anorexia, one would not expect these individuals to become ketotic, but those who some clinicians may consider meet the criteria for EDNOS may well have recurrent DKA, although the evidence for this is extremely limited. The problem is that so far eating disorders have proved particularly intractable and difficult to treat in diabetes. It is also possible that other psychiatric disorders maybe implicated[38–40] but the data on these in relation to DKA is limited at the moment.

A further possible cause is that the young person may go through a period of rebellion or rejection of their diabetes. The very process of learning to live with and cope with a life-limiting condition can lead to feelings of resentment and phases of rebellion. These may lead to periods of insulin omission, which are just part of the process of adapting to life with diabetes, especially during adolescence. As a young lady wrote about her life with diabetes, analogizing her diabetes to a package to be carried around at all times,

A few months on, I became sick of being the only person able to see the big parcel in front of me, with all my attention focused on it. I was unable to enjoy what was going on around me. Why *should* I carry it, I asked, but no one would answer. Then I started thinking, if this was how it was going to be, *forever*, I didn't want any more of it.

I tried to put it down, but couldn't. I tried *throwing* it down, but it was attached to me. I then tried every way I could think of to get rid of it: kicking, pushing, even getting my friends to try and pull it away, everything failed. I then tried to totally destroy it, but it was *me* who suffered from the repercussions (Anon).

Occasional insulin omission may be just an oversight, as diabetes is pushed into the background of adolescent life. Forgetting was the most common reason cited by young people for omitting insulin,[41] but this is unlikely to be the cause for frequent, serious DKA.

Given these and other possible causes of insulin omission, attempting to resolve the associated problems can be difficult. A recent systematic review of educational and psychosocial interventions for adolescents with type 1 diabetes located only six studies targeted at this group of patients.[18] Two studies identified by this review[42,43] report on a range of interventions being used, ranging from changing the insulin regimen, to a nurse giving injections, to family therapy. Other approaches that have been tried include more intensive management (CSII pumps), planned admissions to hospital and cognitive behaviour therapy. All that can be definitely said is that these interventions seem to be of real benefit to some individuals, but not all.

It would seem that an important step in resolving recurrent DKA is a multi-disciplinary assessment by person(s) with knowledge or understanding of the individual from a psychosocial perspective. Some approaches have not been considered, or published, such as the identification and treatment of depression and attention deficit hyperactivity disorder, with medication and individual or family therapy. In attempting to resolve recurrent DKA with any of these treatment modalities, it is important that diabetes drops into the background.

Early identification and open discussion about the causation and associated problems is of paramount importance. Prevention of recurrent DKA should also be high on the health care professionals' agenda. Steps that can be easily incorporated into routine care can serve to prevent the emergence of recurrent DKA. We must learn to identify psychopathologies as soon as possible.

- At diagnosis, where adolescent patients experience substantial weight loss, weight gain should be gradual and not excessive, to avoid eating disorders.

- Young people and families should be given opportunities to talk about their feelings and emotional responses at diagnosis and throughout their childhood and adolescence.

- Diabetes teams should try to include either a psychologist or someone with additional training in counselling as an integral member of the team for all young people and their families.

- Provision of continuing ongoing diabetes education must be readily available.

- Early adolescent autonomy and responsibility for care should not be overly encouraged: responsibility should be given to the adolescent at *their* request, *not the parents'* – it should be a gradual process.

- At times there may be a need to take a few steps back when the burden of diabetes becomes too much, especially when other issues (study, peer pressures, romantic relationships, depression etc.) take priority for the adolescent.

- Most importantly, do not lose contact with the adolescent who is experiencing recurrent DKA and other problems. Keep in touch by whatever means possible, phone, fax, e-mail, post, as your support is essential if damage is to be minimized and the individual is to find a way forward.

2.2 Familial Interventions

First, the descriptive literature of the family environment in supporting the young person with diabetes is probably the most extensively researched area on adolescent and childhood diabetes. To provide a means of integrating the very disparate operationalizations used in the research, two dimensions that family researchers, reviewers and theorists have consistently identified will be used. The labels more usually used for these dimensions are *family support* and *family control*. Family support comprises behaviours that foster in an individual feelings of comfort and belonging, and that he or she is basically accepted and approved of as a person by the parents and family. Family control reflects an environment that directs the behaviour of an individual in a manner desirable to the parents, to the power base in the family.[44]

Although the dimension of family support generates inconsistent results in relation to glycated haemoglobin, with roughly equal numbers of cross-sectional studies supporting an association[49,52–58] and failing to support this association,[45,46,59–67] and longitudinal studies also producing mixed results.[23,23,55,63,71] In contrast, most support a significant association between family support and psychological adjustment,[45–49] although two smaller studies report no significant association between family support and adjustment.[50,51] In relation to self-care the literature consistently supports an association,[46,53,54,62,68–73] with no identified studies failing to find an association between some aspect of family support and self-care behaviour. The inconsistent results for family support and glycaemic control are probably a result of its effect being mediated by self-care, whereas other variables have direct effects,[54] such as stress, which may mask the indirect effect of family support in some studies. Despite these results, to date no study has targeted increasing support with the family.

However, family conflict, a concept related to support, has been targeted in a recent intervention programme. The fact this has been done remains curious, given the inconsistent results in the published literature.[55,61,70] with prospective data[71] reporting that changes in conflict were not associated with changes in adherence over the four years of their prospective longitudinal study. This may be a result of conflict over minor issues being common and even normative in adolescence, with some commentators arguing that conflict in the family is essential for the development of young people's interpersonal skills.[74–76] However, it is important to remember that extreme levels of conflict and/or conflicts that remain continually unresolved are likely to disrupt the family and impact on poor control. Therefore, communication and conflict resolution may be a more critical issue as highlighted by Bobrow and colleagues,[77] who examined the interaction between mothers and adolescent daughters with diabetes. However, if conflict resolution is the key problem then interventions designed to provide families with the skills and strategies to resolve conflicts with resulting benefits for the family as a whole and for the management of diabetes would be helpful. One research group has attempted this using Behavioral–Family Systems Therapy (BFST).[78–81] The programme involves four therapy components. (i) Problem-solving training provides families with a behavioural contracting approach to conflict resolution with training in problem definition; generation of alternative solutions; group decision-making, planning, implementation and monitoring of the selected solution and renegotiation or refinement of the ineffective solutions. (ii) Communication skill training includes instructions, feedback, modelling and rehearsal, targeting common parent–adolescent communication problems. (iii) Cognitive restructuring methods were used to identify and change family members' irrational beliefs, attitudes and attributions that may have impeded effective parent adolescent communication and conflict resolution. (iv) Functional and structural family therapy interventions targeted anomalous family systemic characteristics (e.g. weak parental coalitions or cross-generational coalitions) that may have impeded effective problem solving and communication. The psychologists used standard behaviour therapy techniques of instruction, feedback, modelling and rehearsal along with behavioural homework (i.e. encouraging families to practice targeted skills at home). Although the programme resulted in significant improvements in parent–adolescent relationships and adherence, there were no gains in psychological adjustment or metabolic control.[79–81] These mixed results pose more questions than they answer on the role of conflict and diabetes outcomes. All that can be said for certain at the moment is that the research on family conflict continues to generate conflicting, contradictory and confusing results.

Research on the dimension of family control also generates inconsistent results, with some studies reporting a significant association[46,48,49,51,58–62,66,82–84] whilst others do not support an association.[45,46,52,53,55,60,62–65,70,85–90] This inconsistency may be a result of researchers looking for linear effects, when non-linear effects are more probable.[84] Alternatively, the lack of consistency in results may be a consequence of the lack of specificity in the measures of family control measures. Research that has looked at the degree of parental involvement in diabetes care has produced noticeably consistent results. The greater the responsibility for diabetes care activities (e.g. injecting insulin, deciding on insulin dose, remembering to monitor blood glucose values) taken by the adolescent with diabetes, and the less the parental involvement, the worse the control.[5,58,64,66,91–94] More detailed examination of parent and child perceptions of responsibility indicated that where no-one was taking responsibility for diabetes care tasks the young person with diabetes was in worse diabetes control.[95] This handing over of responsibility not only needs to be negotiated and managed, but also needs to match the maturity of the individual and their ability to take responsibility.[7,94]

These hypotheses have now been tested with intervention studies that specifically targeted this process of negotiating responsibility, combined with self-management education.[96–98] These studies have demonstrated that this is an issue that could be readily integrated into normal diabetes care and consultations without increasing diabetes-related conflict, and can be delivered in a group or individual format and support improved glycaemic control and self-care. This approach has now been replicated by a second research group in the UK.[99,100] FACTS (Families, Adolescents and Children's Teamwork Study), developed in response to the need for a family-centred, skills-based education programme without parents and their children having to attend the hospital for any more visits. There are three or four families in each group with separate sessions for children (11 years or less) and young people (12–16 years). The sessions are fully integrated into routine clinical care and occur at the diabetes centre on the same day as the child's usual 3 monthly appointment. There are four sessions per year, which allows time to consolidate new information and put it into practice before new topics are raised. This approach also helps to include those who may not otherwise volunteer for extra-curricular activities or find attending for additional visits difficult. Each session is facilitated by a health care professional who has had expert training in the delivery of group education by a health psychologist. This has enabled a structured programme to be delivered by local staff while making effective use of the limited health psychologist resources available in the UK.

Session 1 (Food enjoyment with carbohydrate counting) is facilitated by a paediatric diabetes specialist dietitian. Carbohydrate counting is not presented as an all or nothing tool, or as a tool exclusively for those on pumps or multiple injections, but rather as a tool that those on less intensive insulin regimes may also wish to consider. We use real foods eaten by the children and focus on snacks, which contribute significantly to the calorie intake of young people taken either as treats, before sports or to prevent/treat hypos.

To establish what carbohydrate counting is all about and how it may be useful the group is asked what is already known about this topic. They discuss why they feel this may be of benefit in managing diabetes. Once the group has identified that carbohydrate counting may be helpful to them, the next step is for them to identify which foods contain carbohydrate. These are listed on a flip chart and divided into two columns to distinguish sugars and starches as shown. This allows for discussion and recognition of the different types of sugar, e.g. fructose, lactose, sucrose and glucose.

The children write what they have eaten for breakfast that morning on a flip chart. They identify the carbohydrate sources and discuss how these may be counted by using food labels, weighing or using handy measures to work out their portion size. Food reference tables are introduced and used as required. Children are encouraged to choose their favourite snacks from a variety of healthy and sweeter options and work out which ones are suitable snacks. The fact that 15g of carbohydrate has the same effect on blood sugar whether it comes from an apple, a Shredded Wheat or a mini Mars bar is of great interest to the children. The use of snacks before sports and to treat/prevent hypos is discussed.

The practicalities of estimating the carbohydrate content of individual portions of rice or pasta are discussed. The carbohydrate content of 100 g dry basmati rice is calculated and compared to the cooked portion. Families work together to read the labels, weigh their portion and work out the carbohydrate content of their own portion size. They are introduced to handy measures to avoid this messy process at each meal! Those who wish to continue with this at home are given food diaries and asked to calculate their average daily CHO intake. Computer analysis of their results revealed that this simple practical session resulted in effective estimation of CHO content with minimal differences between computer and parent estimates. This indicates that carbohydrate counting can be effectively taught in small groups using real life examples and practical interactive activities. The session is effective in providing accurate dietary knowledge but of course this does not prove that it results in improved insulin dose adjustment or lasting behavioural change.

Session 2 (Blood sugar testing, HbA1c and insulin dose adjustment) builds on the carbohydrate counting session through initially reviewing learning from the first session and the group's experiences with carbohydrate counting with all efforts praised, followed by an outline of the current session contents. Thereafter, a card game is played to explore the facts and fictions of blood sugar monitoring. Individuals are encouraged to think about their own blood glucose targets and comment on how easy or difficult these are to achieve. Factors that raise and lower blood glucose are written on a flip chart, with an emphasis that although food is important it is not the only factor leading to out of range values.

Parents and children are asked whether they know what their HbA1c value was at today's clinic visit. Those who wish to share their results are asked what this means to them in terms of blood sugar control. A practical demonstration follows where the children pour a small amount of granulated sugar into a clear container and a larger amount of sugar into the next. Red blood cells are simulated by making small balls of red playdough, demonstrating that at greater sugar concentrations there is more sugar stuck to the red cells, giving higher levels of HbA1c.

Basic facts about common types of insulin and injection techniques are discussed. Participants are asked to find the names of their own insulins and with help from their parents match these to the time frame over which they work using sticky labels on the flip chart. This simple exercise always reveals a surprising number of common misconceptions. Insulin absorption from different sites and the need for site rotation are discussed.

A pattern of high blood sugars before the evening meal is written on the flip chart. Participants are then asked to come forward and circle those values that are out of range such that they can identify the pattern. The group discusses the likely causes for this pattern. They then suggest a range of solutions, which are offered to each child/young person, who then determines which one will work best for them. Regular review of diaries or blood glucose memories is encouraged at home to encourage parents to elicit their child's opinions and to gain confidence in problem solving as a team.

Session 3 (Teamwork and communication to support blood glucose monitoring) begins with an ice-breaker exercise as the topic moves away from more traditional education to more psychological issues. The group is asked to arrange themselves in order of height with eyes closed, or they are asked hold hands in a circle, drop hands, hold hands with two different people, while staying in same spot and then go back to your original position. Once the task is completed the group is asked 'What did you need to do?'. The answers are written onto the flipchart and form the basis of this session:

'teamwork'

'getting out of a mess'

'rely on someone else to co-operate'

'have a laugh'

'getting to know people'

'how to work out a problem with each other'

'trust each other'

'there are lots of solutions', 'always a way out'

'cannot always get it perfect'.

Thereafter children and parents are both asked to draw a picture of doing a blood sugar test in their home. They are encouraged to share their pictures with the group:

Michael (grumpy face) – Please do I have to?

Mum – Yes.

Michael – Can I do it later?

Mum – It's always come on, come on, come on until in the end I get a grumpy face too. Once he starts doing it, it's OK.

After sharing these pictures and describing what is happening, the group are to draw 'what happens in your house when your blood sugar is 22.5'. This provides an opportunity to discuss how families react to out of range blood glucose values. The issues raised by this are discussed, with many parents and children gaining new insights into each other's behaviours and how these affect each other's feelings and thoughts about themselves. Throughout, no one is criticized or judged; rather, individuals views are all valued and everyone is just given time to share their views in an honest but gentle way.

Session 4 (Interdependence: sharing responsibility and letting go) also begins with another ice breaking exercise, before asking the group to 'Draw a train representing your diabetes team'. Everyone is again gently persuaded to share their drawings, and some specific questions are asked of both adolescents and parents, such as 'Who's driving the trian?'; 'In which carriage do you sit?'; 'How do you feel about where you are?'; 'How can you see this changing in the future?'; 'What needs to happen to help these changes happen?'.

There tends to be more agreement between the pictures drawn by the parents and adolescents in this session, compared to session 3, but here the discussion is focused on the future, and negotiating changing roles as the young person gets older. Any key points raised in the discussion are noted on a flip chart. There is no direct teaching or instruction in the session, just valuing the insights brought to the group by the participants.

The FACTS programme aims to improve diabetes self-management skills, increase teamwork and reduce diabetes-related family conflict. A randomized waiting-list-controlled trial is currently underway to assess the effects of the programme on quality of life and glycaemic control of young people with type 1 diabetes. The preliminary data from this project are promising. With more families attending the group requesting to go on more intensive insulin regimens, although this is not the aim of the educators, the intervention group show increased agreement between parents and adolescents on diabetes management tasks, more adolescent and more parental involvement in care and improved glycaemic control in the short term.

The results of these studies replicates the data on general adolescent development, which also implicates parental involvement as the single most important predictor of positive adolescent outcomes.[101] The key to understanding this approach is to acknowledge that the major developmental task of adolescence is movement away from dependence on the family, not toward complete independence but rather interdependence. Interdependence does not require the adolescents to distance themselves emotionally from parents, but requires a reorganization in which the family members renegotiate and redistribute responsibilities and obligations.

2.3 Individual Interventions

Despite the benefits of these family-based programmes, they pose a challenge for working with older adolescents if their parents do not come to clinic or for young people in families who are not supportive of their diabetes care, and so may not want to attend for these sessions. Possibly as a result of these drives there has been a growth in a number of programmes designed for adolescents. The programme with the longest pedigree and most robust evidence here is the work of Grey and colleagues.[102–104] They have evaluated the impact of a coping skills training programme as an adjunct for adolescents starting intensive insulin regimens, either multiple daily injections or continuous subcutaneous insulin infusion. The aim of the programme is to increase adolescents' sense of competence and mastery by giving training in positive coping skills for the stresses arising from intensive management. Specifically, the programme taught social problem solving, social, cognitive behaviour modification and conflict resolution skills using scenarios that the adolescent generated as causing problems for intensive management. The programme used a professional educator for the first few group sessions, and then moved on to using a trained adolescent with diabetes to complete the programme. The results of the programme, evaluated using a randomized trial, are very encouraging, showing improved glycaemic control and psychological outcomes in the short term, which were sustained at 1 year follow-up. However, the challenge here is that this programme is designed for adolescents on intensive insulin regimens, and so may be a useful adjunct to the process of starting adolescents on intensive regimens, but restricts the applicability of this approach to all adolescents with diabetes, many of whom will be on less intensive regimens (e.g. twice a day injections).

Therefore, approaches for individuals need to be considered to provide a more productive approach. Howells and colleagues explore this approach,[105] using regular telephone calls, every 2–3 weeks, designed to provide support and assistance in using problem-solving steps: define the problem; set a realistic goal for change; brainstorm – generate likely solutions; decide which solution to try; plan, act and review. Participants were at liberty to choose the subject of the call. They were informed that diabetes management did not have to be a focus for discussion, and the calls were not used to feed back HbA1c results. Although the intervention groups showed improvements in self-efficacy this was not matched by improvements in glycaemic control. Process analysis indicated that barriers to insulin use was a strong predictor of glycaemic control. This suggests that using this approach but focusing content on issues related to diabetes management, as in Grey's group programme, as well as other non-diabetes issues may be needed to show an effect on metabolic outcomes.

A second approach that is gaining increasing attention for adolescents in this area is the use of motivational interviewing.[106] Motivational interviewing (MI) has been described as a directive, counselling style for eliciting behaviour change by helping clients to explore and resolve ambivalence.[107,108] MI has been implemented in a variety of health care settings within adult populations. The results from two systematic reviews[109,110] have found impressive effect sizes (0.33 and above) for studies delivering MI in substance misuse. The results are less conclusive for other lifestyle areas. In the published research with teenagers and MI, most studies have been in the substance misuse field,[111,112] with some pilot studies demonstrating positive results in the diabetes field.[106,113,114]

Using MI with teenagers who have diabetes seems to make sense as there is an intuitive fit with the central tenets of MI such as rapport building, directiveness and empathy, which are central to care of adolescents with type 1 diabetes. A major step in engaging adolescents in care is to gain their trust, and the 'spirit' of MI involves the collaboration between client and practitioner; supporting autonomy and conveying respect for the adolescent is particularly appealing in engaging young people. The central tenet of ambivalence presents a key challenge in the clinical care of adolescents. Although many young people are resilient and experience no problems with diabetes, there will be just as many who will have a turbulent time with achieving optimal glycaemic control. Furthermore, the dynamics between health care provider and young person can often reflect conflicts in the adolescents' world.

The promise that MI theory and pilot studies have suggested has recently been tested in a randomized controlled trial of MI with adolescents, using the core strategies or tools outlined in Table 2.1. To address the criticism of MI literature that there is a lack of scientific evaluation of the methods used,[115,116] and issues relating to interventionist training, supervision and quality monitoring, the study used direct clinical supervision. Furthermore, to provide a more rigorous test of the MI, individuals randomized to the control group received supportive counselling from a diabetes nurse specialist.

At 12 months significant differences were found, with MI participants reporting higher life satisfaction and lower life worry, less anxiety and more positive well-being. The intervention group also held a higher belief in controlling for their diabetes, a higher belief that certain actions were more likely to help prevent future complications of diabetes, a higher perception that their diabetes had a small degree of impact on their lives and a higher perception of seriousness of their diabetes than controls. These changes resulted in meaningful and significant improvement in glycaemic control at 24 months follow-up.[117] Alternatively, the MI intervention may also activate the individual to be more pro-active in their diabetes management, as the change in illness beliefs would suggest, but unless they have the optimal regimen for their lifestyle and or have the requisite skills for insulin dose adjustment these motivational changes may not result in changes in metabolic markers.

Although the MI work so far with adolescents with diabetes, is only showing promise, some of the tools utilized from the menu in Table 2.1 are worth considering in more detail, as they seem to share much with other intervention programmes and can be used within a diverse range of theoretical models.

Table 2.1   Motivation interviewing with adolecents' menu of strategies

- Setting the scene
- Agenda setting task
- Typical day
- Pros and cons
- Importance, confidence and readiness
- Significant others
- The journey of change
- Perspectives of young person with diabetes
- Exploring concerns
- Goals and action

Pros and cons

First, adolescents may often have conflicting feelings, attitudes and thoughts about changing their behaviour, particularly if the behaviour is habitual, entrenched, and has personal valence. One useful tool is to look at the positives and negatives of current behaviour and of change. The strategy aims to provide structure, raise awareness and elicit thoughts and feelings about current behaviour. This is an exercise that will be familiar from other approaches and can seem to be a simple exercise. However, it needs to be carried out slowly and sensitively, with respect for the patient's decisions on how they value their behaviour(s). It is in this exercise that the adolescent's fairly fragile sense of their independent self can become very apparent and impact on the process. For this to be a productive exercise the young person must have developed a significant degree of trust in the counsellor to believe that his or her perspective will not be discounted. Virtually all other people in the person's life have a vested interest in hearing him or her talk in a particular way about behaviour. Without trust the exercise becomes a recital of risks to health which, whilst they may motivate some, may not be the crucial ingredient of change for many. This may be the first time adolescents with diabetes may have faced their 'dilemmas' and spoken about them honestly. The power of ambivalence will become particularly marked in this exercise and the counsellor must work extremely hard to use this constructively before less constructive alternatives are adopted to reduce the dissonance.

In order to appreciate the dilemmas young people face and to start to understand the decisions they make, it is important to understand and explore their frame of reference for their diabetes management. Perception of illness shape how the young person copes with, controls and adheres to the illness and plays a central role in outcomes.[118] Personal illness models[119–121] are identified as patients' cognitive representations, which will impact distally on illness-related behaviour. These representations include the degree to which a person can control the illness, the cause of illness, how long the illness endures and the consequences of illness.[122] Assessing degree of perception of control may be of particular importance with diabetes, for which glycaemic control is significant in preventing complications.

Some adolescents will keep a tight rein on their diabetes management and will practice health-affirming behaviours to keep their diabetes management within normal limits. Others will be happy to hand over responsibility to their treatment regimen and significant others. However, diabetes is a complex metabolic disorder, and for some young people tight control, perfect lifestyle factors and supportive families do not always equal positive outcomes. Puberty has negative pharmacological effects on secretion of insulin[123] and this will have a profound effect on their management.

Process of change

Diabetes poses considerable demands on the young person's coping, self-esteem, mood and quality of life. Once a decision has been taken to change, then implementing the desired behaviour depends on several factors. A taxonomy of conflicting goals will be occurring in the young person's social circle, thinking and behaviours. Although a young person may shrug off the complexities of for example increasing the frequency of injecting insulin from twice daily to four times daily, complex intra- and inter-personal processes will be guiding the young person in adopting novel behaviours.

One strategy that has been used and received very positively by adolescents was voicing commitment to change, by discussing 'the journey of change'. It is a genuine attempt at understanding how the young person adapts to and copes with change in all different areas of their life, e.g. learning a new sport or musical instrument, coping with exams etc. This hopefully enables them to reflect on their strengths and previous successes and failures. Again, the aim is to put diabetes in the context of other aspects of their life in a constructive way.

This strategy attempts to examine the underlying *how* of the change trajectory based on the idea, formulated by Bandura,[124] that people cannot influence their motivation and actions very well if they do not pay adequate attention to their own performances, the conditions under which they occur and the immediate and distal effects they produce. The strategy taps into the self-regulatory notion of volition or *trying*[125,126] by unpacking the processes of goal progress monitoring and efficacy coping, to understand how the young person overcomes implementation problems such as putting goals into practice. It is an attempt to understand and reflect on the young persons' 'how' of adapting to change, compared with the 'what' they are going to change. In making these processes tangible, the young persons are able to examine their own barriers to change, successes they have experienced and how they maintain their patterns of behaviour and also prevent relapse.

Part of the discussion of previous experiences of change will include the role that other people have played in facilitating or impeding the process. Discussing their preference for a 'coach', 'teacher' or 'parent' alongside them will help them think about what they need to help them move on and specifically the nature of the relationship with the counsellor. This collaborative strategy needs to be implemented when trust and rapport have become established, and when the young person is voicing commitment to change. It can facilitate problem solving and goal planning, and build on confidence.

Importance, confidence and readiness

A core strategy of MI incorporates the concepts of importance, confidence and readiness.[127] The assessments of these values are presented on linear scales of gradations between 0 to 10 (with 10 being the highest value). Miller and Rollnick[108] suggest that the importance or personal valence of changing must be explored against the ability or confidence to change. The underlying principles tap into self-regulatory theories such as Bandura's[128,129] self-efficacy model, and the theory of reasoned action of Ajzen and Fishbein.[130] The health action process model of Schwarzer and Fuch[126] offers health cognitions analogous to these dimensions (with importance paralleling outcome expectancies and confidence paralleling efficacy beliefs).[129] The distinctions between the three constructs are useful heuristics and have practical applicability in consultations. Rollnick *et al.*[127] argue that having established a numerical value for the person's values, this sets the stage for the person thinking hard about change. It also helps the counsellor consider with the client the nature and focus of their involvement. If a professional asks a young person how important it is to them to make a particular change and how confident he or she is (using a 0–10 scale) then this can be used to inform how to take things forward. For example, a score of nine on importance and three on confidence should lead to a discussion that will be focussed on building confidence. If the scores are reversed, then motivation to change is low so exploring the pros and cons of change might be the way forward, or it may be best to concentrate on other areas of change first.

Goals and action

Once change has been decided upon, the next step is to slowly and constructively develop a plan for change. The counsellor steers the process with maximal patient autonomy. It is beneficial to draw on the experiences of change plans from other adolescents in the study and what has/has not worked for them. This allows social comparison with peers and assessment of their own beliefs and sense of efficacy. It requires careful thought on the part of the adolescent as any goals set should be realistic, achievable within a short time span, measurable and evaluative. Thus, a certain degree of help is required in negotiating a suitable and workable plan. The young persons may still have some conflicting feelings about change, and it is important to respect their wishes and difficulties, working at their own pace. Working with teenagers will occasionally bring the counsellor into consideration of risk behaviours, particularly as part of the teenager's social interaction, which brings with it its own ethical dilemmas.

2.4   Conclusion

Over the last decade there has been a trend in the adolescent literature to focus more on intervention studies. Furthermore, these studies seem to have responded to the criticisms in the published reviews, with most articulating a clear theoretical rationale for their intervention methods, and predominantly using randomized trial designs. The value of supporting parents and adolescents to negotiate their way through issues around the transfer of diabetes care responsibility continues to receive support. This work can be done in small groups, or with individual families, and positive results have now been demonstrated by two independent research teams. Interventions with individual adolescents have also continued to develop. Where the intervention has targeted the specific needs of a specific population, those starting on intensive insulin regimens, the results have been very positive. However, generic approaches continue to produce results that show trends toward positive effects, but the studies would appear to be underpowered. Clearly there is a need for more multi-centre working on these generic approaches, if large enough samples are to be secured to generate robust results. The one thing that does continue to be consistent throughout this literature is that many of the programmes, either explicitly or implicitly, use approaches that are designed to enhance self-efficacy. Therefore, for health care professionals, understanding the role of self-efficacy or confidence and how to support it would seems to be one key to productive working relationships with adolescents and young people with diabetes.

However, it is important to remember that the techniques to develop self-efficacy (mastery experience, modelling, verbal persuasion and emotion regulation) are not sufficient to facilitate change. For these techniques, or any other psychological educational intervention, to work, they must be accompanied by appropriate attitudes and qualities from the professional. The simplest way to summarize these qualities is acceptance (of the person, regardless of their behaviour and beliefs), respect (for each individual's decision; everyone makes the best decision they can to optimize their quality of life, given *their* perception of *their* situation), curiosity (to genuinely understand the world the young persons live in, their thoughts and feelings, which drive their decisions) and honesty (about what you as a professional think and feel, and why you hold the beliefs you do). In many if not all therapeutic relationships these qualities are more important than particular techniques or strategies used by the professional, and these should be a priority for professional development.

References

1. Wysocki T, Clarke WL, Meinhold PA, Bellando BJ, Abrams EC, Bourgeois MJ, Barnard MU. Parental and professional estimates of self-care independence of children and adolescents with IDDM. *Diabetes Care* 1992; **15** (1): 43–52.
2. Ingersoll GM, Orr DP, Herrold AJ, Golden MP. Cognitive maturity and self-management among adolescents with insulin-dependent diabetes mellitus. *J Pediatr* 1986; **108**: 620–623.
3. Allen DA, Tennen H, McGrade BJ, Affleck G, Ratzan S. Parent and child perceptions of the management of juvenile diabetes. *J Pediatr Psychol* 1983; **8** (2): 129–141.
4. Mortensen HB, Villumsen J, Volund A, Petersen KE, Nerup J. The Danish Study Group of Diabetes in Childhood. Relationship between insulin injections regimen and metabolic control in young Danish type 1 diabetic patients. *Diabet Med* 1992; **9**: 834–9.
5. Jacobson AM, Hauser ST, Lavori P, Willett JB, Cole CF, Wolfsdorf JI, Dumont RH, Wertileb D. Family environment and glycemic control: a four-year prospective study of children and adolescnts with insulin-dependent diabetes mellitus. *Psychosomat Med* 1994; **56**: 401–409.
6. Hoey H, Mortensen H, McGee H, Fitzgeralt M. Hvidøre Group. Is metabolic control related to quality of life? A study of 2103 children and adolescents with IDDM from 17 countries. *Diabetes Res Clin Practice* 1999; **44** (Suppl.): S3.
7. Amiel SA, Sherwin RS, Simonson DC, Lauritano AA, Tamborland WV. Impaired insulin action in puberty: a contributing factor to poor glycemic control in adolescents with diabetes. *N Eng J Med* 1986; **315**: 215–9.
8. Hindmarsh PC, Matthews SG, Silvio LDI. Relations between height velocity and fasting insulin concentrations. *Arch Dis Child* 1988; **63**: 666.
9. Johnson SB, Kelly M, Henretta JC, Cunningham WR, Tomer A, Silverstein JH. A longitudinal analysis of adherence and health status in childhood diabetes. *J Pediatr Psychol* 1992; **17** (5): 537–553.
10. Johnson SB, Silverstein J, Rosenbloom A, Carter R, Cunningham W. Assessing daily management of childhood diabetes. *Health Psychol* 1986; **9**: 545–564.
11. Morris AD, Boyle DIR, McMahon AD, Greene SA, MacDonald TM, Newton RW. Adherence to insulin treatment, glycemic control and ketoacidosis in insulin-dependent diabetes mellitus. *Lancet* 1997; **350**: 1505–1510.

12. Thompson CJ, Greene SA. Diabetes in the older teenager and young adult. In Court S, Lamb B (eds), *Childhood and Adolescent Diabetes*. London: Wiley, 1997, pp 67–76.

13. Elleman K. Soerensen JN. Pedesen L. Edsberg B, Andersen OO. Epidemiology and treatment of diabetic ketoacidosis in a community population. *Diabetes Care* 1984; **7**: 528–532.

14. Olsen R, Sutton J. More hassle, more alone: adolescents with diabetes and the role of formal and informal support. *Child: Care, Health Dev* 1998; **24** (1): 31–39.

15. Griffin SJ. Lost to follow-up: the problem of defaulters from diabetes clinics. *Diabet Med* 1998; **15** (Suppl. 3): S14–S24.

16. Steel JM, Young RJ, Lloyd GG *et al*. Abnormal eating attitudes in young insulin dependent diabetics. *Br J Psychiatry* 1989; **155**: 515–521.

17. Neumark-Sztainer D, Story M, Toporoff E, Himes JH, Resnick MD, Blum RWM. Covariations of eating behaviors with other health-related behaviors among adolescents. *J Adolescent Health* 1997; **20**: 450–458.

18. Hampson SE, Skinner TC, Hart J, Storey L, Gage H, Foxcroft D, Kimber A, Shaw K, Walker J. Effects of educational and psychosocial interventions for adolescents with diabetes mellitus: a systematic review. *Health Technol Assessment* 2001; **5** (10).

19. Gage H, Hampson S, Skinner TC, Hart J, Storey L, Foxcroft D, Kimber A, Cradock S, McEvilly EA. Educational and psychosocial programmes for adolescents with diabetes: approaches, outcomes and cost-effectiveness. *Patient Education Counselling* 2004; **53** (3): 333–346.

20. Hampson SE, Skinner TC, Hart J, Storey L, Gage H, Foxcroft D, Kimber A, Cradock S, McEvilly AE. Behavioral interventions for adolescents with type 1 diabetes: how effective are they? *Diabetes Care* 2000; **23** (9): 1416–1422.

21. Laing SP, Swerdlow AJ, Slater SD, Botha JL, Burden AC, Waugh NR, Smith AWM, Hill RD, Bingley PJ, Patterson CC, Qiao Z, Keen H. The British Diabetic Association Cohort Study, II: Cause specific mortality in patients with insulin-treated diabetes mellitus. *Diab Med* 1999; **16**: 471.

22. Kovacs M, Charron-Prochownik D, Obrosky DS. A longitudinal study of biomedical and psychosocial predictors of multiple hospitalizations among young people with insulin-dependent diabetes mellitus. *Diab Med* 1995; **12**: 142–148.

23. Herskowitz RD, Jacobson AM, Cole C, Hauser ST, Wolfsdorf JI, Willett JB, Milley JE, Wertileb D. Psychosocial predictors of acute complications of diabetes in youth. *Diab Med* 1995; **12**: 612–618.

24. Tattersall RB. Brittle diabetes revisited: The Third Arnold Bloom Memorial Lecture. *Diab Med* 1997; **14**: 99–110.

25. Tattersall RB, Gregory R, Selby C, Kerr D, Heller S. Course of brittle diabetes: 12 year follow up. *BMJ* 1991; **302**: 1240–1243.

26. Kent LA, Gill GV, Williams G. Mortality and outcome of patients with brittle diabetes and recurrent ketoacidosis. *Lancet* 1994; **344**: 778–781.

27. White K, Kolman ML, Wexler P, Polin G, Winter RJ. Unstable diabetes and unstable families: a psychosocial evaluation of diabetic children with recurrent ketoacidosis. *Pediatrics* 1984; **73**: 749–755.

28. Rosen H, Lidz T. Emotional factors in the precipitation of recurrent diabetic ketoacidosis. *Psychosom Med* 1949; **11**: 211–215.

29. Liss DS, Waller DA, Kennard BD, McIntire D, Capra P, Stephens J. Psychiatric illness and family support in children and adolescents with diabetic ketoacidosis: a controlled study. *J Am Acad Child Adol Psych* 1998; **37**: 536–544.

30. Peveler RC, Bryden KS, Neil HA, Fairburn CG, Mayou RA, Dunger DB, Turner HM. The relationship of disordered eating habits and attitudes to clinical outcomes in young adult females with type 1 diabetes. *Diabetes Care* 2005; **28** (1): 84–88.

31. Engstrom I, Kroon M, Arvidsson CG, Segnestam K, Snellman K, Aman J. Eating disorder in adolescent girls with insulin-dependent diabetes mellitus: a population-based case-control study. *Acta Paediatr* 1999; **88**: 175–180.
32. Stancin T, Link DL, Reuter JM. Binge eating and purging in young women with IDDM. *Diabetes Care* 1989; **12** (9): 601–603.
33. Rodin GM, Daneman D, Johnson LE, Kenshole A. Garfinkel P. Anorexia and bulimia in female adolescents with insulin dependent diabetes mellitus: a systematic study. *J Psychiat Res* 1985; **19** (2): 381–384.
34. Peveler RC, Fairburn CG, Boller I, Dunger D. Eating disorders in adolescents with IDDM: a controlled study. *Diabetes Care* 1992; **15** (10): 1356–1360.
35. Bryden KS, Peveler RC, Neil A, Fairburn CG, Mayou RA, Dunger DB. Eating habits, body weight and insulin misuse: a longitudinal study of teenagers and young adults with type 1 diabetes. *Diabetes Care* 1999; **22** (12): 1956–1960.
36. Striegal-Moore RH, Nicholson TJ, Tamborlane WV. Prevalence of eating disorder symptoms in preadolescent and adolescent girls with IDDM. *Diabetes Care* 1992; **15** (10): 1361–1368.
37. Jones JM, Lawson ML, Daneman D, Olmsted MP, Rodin G. Eating disorders in adolescent females with and without type 1 diabetes: cross sectional study. *BMJ* 2000; **320** (7249): 1563–1566.
38. Blanz BJ, Rensch-Riemann BS, Fritz-Sigmund DI, Schmidt MH. IDDM is a risk factor for adolescent psychiatric disorders. *Diabetes Care* 1993; **16** (12): 1579–1587.
39. Kovacs M, Ho V, Pollock MH. Criterion and predictive validity of the diagnosis of adjustment disorder: a prospective study of youths with new-onset insulin-dependent diabetes mellitus. *Am J Psychiatry* 1995; **152**: 523–528.
40. Northam EA, Matthews LK, Anderson PJ, Cameron FJ, Werther GA. Psychiatric morbidity and health outcome in Type 1 diabetes–perspectives from a prospective longitudinal study. *Diabet Med* 2005; **22** (2): 152–157.
41. Weissberg-Benchel J, Wirtz P, Glasgow AM, Turek J, Tynan WD, Ward J. Adolescent diabetes management and mismanagement. *Diabetes Care* 1995; **18**: 77–82.
42. Golden MP, Herrold AJ, Orr DP. An approach to prevention of recurrent diabetic ketoacidosis in the pediatric population. *J Pediatr* 1985; **107**: 195–200.
43. Chase HP, Rose B, Hoops S, Archer PG, Cribari JM. Techniques for improving glucose control in type I diabetes. *Pediatrician* 1985; **12**: 229–235.
44. Maccoby E, Martin J. Socialization on the context of the family: parent–child interaction. In Heatherington E (ed.), *Mussen Manual of Child Psychology.* Vol. 4. 4th edn. New York: Wiley, 1983, pp 1–102.
45. Overstreet S, Goins J, Chen RS, Holmes CS, Greer T, Dunlap WP, Frentz J. Family environment and the interrealtion of family structure, child behavior and metabolic control for children with diabetes. *J Pediatr Psychol* 1995; **20** (4): 435–447.
46. Hanson CL, Henggeler SW, Harris MA, Mitchell KA, Carle DL, Burghen GA. Associations between family members' perceptions of the health care system and the health of youths with insulin-dependent diabetes mellitus. *J Pediatr Psychol* 1988; **13** (4): 543–554.
47. Safyer AW, Hauser ST, Jacobson AM, Bliss R, Herskowitz RD, Wolfsdorf JI, Wertileb D. The impact of the family on diabetes adjustment: a developmental perspective. *Child Adolescent Social Work J* 1993; **10** (2): 123–140.
48. Wertileb D, Hauser ST, Jacobson AM. Adaptation to diabetes: behavior symptoms and family context. *J Pediatr Psychol* 1986; **11** (4): 463–479.
49. Wysocki T. Associations among teen–parent relationships, metabolic control, and adjustment to diabetes in adolescents. *J Pediatr Psychol* 1993; **18** (4): 441–452.

50. Varni JW, Babani L, Wallander JL, Roe TF, Fraiser SD. Social support and self-esteem effects on psychological adjustment in children and adolescents with insulin-dependent diabetes mellitus. *Child Family Behavior Ther* 1989; **11** (1): 1–17.

51. Hauser SM, Jacobson AM, Wertileb D, Brink S, Wentworth S. The contribution of family environment to perceived competence and illness adjustment in diabetic and acutely ill adolescents. *Family Relations* 1985; **34**: 99–108.

52. Anderson BJ, Miller JP, Auslander WF, Santiago JV. Family characteristics of diabetic adolescents: relationship to metabolic control. *Diabetes Care* 1981; **4** (6): 586–594.

53. Burroughs TE, Pontious SL, Santiago JV. The relationship among six psychosocial domains, age, health care adherence, and metabolic control in adolescents with IDDM. *Diabetes Educator* 1993; **19** (5): 396–402.

54. Hanson CL, Schinkel AM, De Guire MJ, Kolterman OG. Empirical validation for a family-centered model of care. *Diabetes Care* 1995; **18** (10): 1347–1356.

55. Auslander WF, Anderson BA, Bubb J, Jung KC, Santiago JV. Risk factors to health in diabetic children: a prospective study from diagnosis. *Health Social Work* 1990; **15** (2): 133–142.

56. Marteau TM, Bloch S, Baum JD. Family life and diabetic control. *J Clin Psychol Psychiatry* 1987; **28** (6): 823–833.

57. Hansson K, Ryden O, Johnsson P. Parent-rated family climate: a concomitant to metabolic control in juvenile IDDM? *Family Syst Med* 1994; **12** (4): 405–413.

58. Waller DA, Chipman JJ, Hardy BW, Hightower MS, North AJ, Williams SB, Babick AJ. Measuring diabetes-specific family support and its relation to metabolic control: a preliminary report. *J Am Acad Child Psychiatry* 1986; **25**: 415–418.

59. Evans CL, Hughes IA. The relationship between diabetic control and individual and family characteristics. *J Psychosomat Res* 1987; **31** (3): 367–374.

60. Burns KL, Green P, Chase HP. Psychosocial correlates of glycemic control as a function of age in youth with insulin-dependent diabetes. *J Adolescent Health* 1986; **7**: 311–319.

61. Weist MD, Finney JW, Barnard MU, Davis CD, Ollendick TH. Empirical selection of psychosocial treatment targets for children and adolescents with diabetes. *J Pediatr Psychol* 1993; **18** (1): 11–28.

62. Schafer LC, Glasgow RE, McCaul KD, Dreher M. Adherence to IDDM regimens: relationship to psychosocial variables and metabolic control. *Diabetes Care* 1983; **6** (5): 493–498.

63. Seiffge-Krenke I. The highly structured climate in families of adolescents with diabetes: functional or dysfunctional for metabolic control. *J Pediatr Psychol* 1998; **23** (5): 313–322.

64. Gowers SG, Jones JC, Kiana S, North CD, Price DA. Family functioning: a correlate of diabetic control? *J Child Psychol Psychiatry* 1995; **36** (6): 993–1001.

65. Kovacs M, Kass RE, Schnell TM, Goldston D, Marsh J. Family functioning and metabolic control of school-aged children with IDDM. *Diabetes Care* 1989; **12** (6): 409–414.

66. McKelvey J, Waller DA, North AJ, Marks JF, Schreiner B, Travis LB, Murphy JN. Reliability and validity of the Diabetes Family Behavior Scale (DFBS). *Diabetes Educator* 1993; **19** (2): 125–132.

67. Pendley JS, Kasmen LJ, Miller DL, Donze J, Swenson C, Reeves G. Peer and family support in children and adolescents with type 1 diabetes. *J Pediatr Psychol* 27 (5).

68. Palardy N, Greening L, Ott J, Holderby A, Atchison J. Adolescents' health attitudes and adherence to treatment for insulin-dependent diabetes mellitus. *Dev Behav Pediatr* 1998; **19** (1): 31–37.

69. McCaul KD, Glasgow RE, Schafer LC. Diabetes regimen behaviour: predicting adherence. *Med Care* 1987; **25** (9): 868–881.

70. Miller-Johnson S, Emery RE, Marvin RS, Clarke W, Lovinger R, Martin M. Parent–child relationships and the management of insulin-dependent diabetes mellitus. *J Consult Clin Psychol* 1994; **62** (3): 603–610.

71. Hauser SM, Jacobson AM, Lavori P, Wolfsdorf JI, Herskowitz RD, Milley JE, Bliss R. Adherence among children and adolescents with insulin-dependent diabetes mellitus over a four-year longitudinal follow-up: II. Immediate and long-term linkages with family milieu. *J Pediatr Psychol* 1990; **15** (4): 527–542.

72. Kyngas H, Hentinen M, Barlow JH. Adolescents' perceptions of physicians, nurses, parents and friends: help or hindrance in compliance with diabetes self-care? *Journal* 1998; **27**: 760–769.

73. La Greca AM, Auslander WF, Greco P, Spetter D, Fisher EB, Santiago JV. I get by with a little help from my family and friends: adolescents' support for diabetes care. *J Pediatr Psychol* 1995; **20** (4): 449–476.

74. Noller P, Callan V. *The Adolescent in the Family*. London: Routledge, 1991.

75. Grotevant HD, Copper CR. Individuality and connectedness in adolescent development: review and prospects for research on identity, relationships and context. In Skoe E, von der Lippe A (eds), *Personality Development in Adolescence* London: Routledge, 1998.

76. von der Lippe A. Are conflict and challenge sources of personality development? Ego development and family communications. In Skoe E, von der Lippe A (eds), *Personality Development in Adolescence*. London: Routledge, 1998.

77. Bobrow ES, AvRuskin TW, Siller J. Mother–daughter interaction and adherence to diabetes regimens. *Diabetes Care* 1985; **8** (2): 146–151.

78. Wysocki T, Harris MA, Greco P, Bubb J, Elder-Danda C, Harvey LM, McDonell K, Taylor A, White NH. Randomized, controlled trial of behavior therapy for families of adolescents with insulin dependent diabetes mellitus. *J Pediatr Psychol* 2000; **25**: 23–33.

79. Wysocki T, Miller K, Greco P, Harris MA, Harvey LM, Taylor A, Elder-Danda C, McDonell K, White NH. Behavior therapy for families of adolescents with diabetes: effects on directly observed family interactions. *Behav Ther* 1999; **30**: 507–525.

80. Wysocki T, Greco P, Harris MA, Harvey LM, McDonell K, Elder CL, Bubb J, White NH. Social validity of support group and behavior therapy interventions for families of adolescents with insulin-dependent diabetes mellitus. *J Pediatr Psychol* 1997; **22**: 635–649.

81. Wysocki T, Greco P, Harris MA, Bubb J, White NH. Behavior therapy for families of adolescents with diabetes: maintenance of treatment effects. *Diabetes Care* 2001; **24** (3): 441–446.

82. Hanson CL, Henggeler SW, Harris MA, Burghen GA, Moore M. Family systems variables and the health status of adolescents with insulin-dependent diabetes mellitus. *Health Psychol* 1989; **8** (2): 239–253.

83. McKelvey J, Waller DA, Stewart SM, Kennard BD, North AJ, Chipman JJ. Family support for diabetes: a pilot study for measuring disease-specific behaviours. *Child Health Care* 1989; **18** (1): 37–41.

84. Gustafsson PA, Cederblad M, Ludvigsson J, Lundin B. Family interaction and metabolic balance in juvenile diabetes mellitus: a prospective study. *Diabetes Res Clin Pract* 1987; **4**: 7–14.

85. Auslander WF, Bubb J, Rogge M, Santiago JV. Family stress and resources: potential areas of intervention in children recently diagnosed with diabetes. *Health Social Work* 1993; **18** (2): 101–113.

86. Wysocki T. Associations among teen–parent relationships, metabolic control, and adjustment to diabetes in adolescents. *J Pediatr Psychol* 1993; **18** (4): 441–452.

87. Jacobson AM, Hauser ST, Lavori P, Willett JB, Cole CF, Wolfsdorf JI, Dumont RH, Wertileb D. Family environment and glycemic control: a four-year prospective study of

children and adolescents with insulin-dependent diabetes mellitus. *Psychosomat Med* 1994; **56**: 401–409.

88. Liss DS, Waller DA, Kennard BD, McIntire D, Capra P, Stephens J. Psychiatric illness and family support in children and adolescents with diabetic ketoacidosis: a controlled study. *J Am Acad Child Adolescent Psychiatry* 1998; **37** (5): 536–544.

89. Hauser SM, Jacobson AM, Lavori P, Wolfsdorf JI, Herskowitz RD, Milley JE, Bliss R. Adherence among children and adolescents with insulin-dependent diabetes mellitus over a four-year longitudinal follow-up: II. Immediate and long-term linkages with family milieu. *J Pediatr Psychol* 1990; **15** (4): 527–542.

90. Bennett Murphy LM, Thompson RJ, Morris MA. Adherence behavior among adolescents with type I insulin-dependent diabetes mellitus: the role of cognitive appraisal processes. *J Pediatr Psychol* 1997; **22**: 811–825.

91. Stevenson K, Sensky T, Petty R. Glycaemic control in adolescents with type I diabetes and parental expressed emotion. *Psychother Psychosomat* 1997; **55**: 170–175.

92. Smith MS, Mauseth R, Palmer JP, Pecoraro R, Wenet G. Glycosyalted hemoglobin and psychological adjustment in adolescents with diabetes. *Adolescence* 1991; **26**: 31–40.

93. La Greca AM, Follansbee D, Skyler JS. Developmental and behavioral aspects of diabetes management in youngsters. *Child Health Care* 1990; **19** (3): 132–139.

94. Wysocki T, Linscheid TR, Taylor AT, Yeates KO, Hough BS, Naglieri JA. Deviation from developmentally appropriate self-care autonomy. *Diabetes Care* 1996; **19** (2): 119–125.

95. Anderson BJ, Auslander WF, Jung KC, Miller JP, Santiago JV, Abraham C, Hampson SE. Assessing family sharing of diabetes responsibilities. *J Pediatr Psychol* 1990; **15** (4): 477–492.

96. Anderson BJ, Joyce H, Brackeyy J, Laffel LMB. An office-based intervention to maintain parent–adolescent teamwork in diabetes management. *Diabetes Care* 1999; **22** (5): 713–721.

97. Anderson BJ, Wolf FM, Bukhart MT, Cornell RG, Bacon GE. Effects of peer-group intervention on metabolic control of adolescents with IDDM: randomized outpatient study. *Diabetes Care* 1989; **12** (3): 179–183.

98. Laffel LMB, Vangsness L, Connell A, Goebel-Fabbri A, Butler D, Anderson BJ. Impact of ambulatory, family-focused teamwork intervention on glycemic control in youth with type 1 diabetes. *J Pediatr* 2003; **142**: 409–416.

99. Murphy HR, Skinner TC, Wadham C, Byard AJ, Rayman G. The Families and Children Teamwork Study (FACTS): recruitment details from a randomized controlled trial of a diabetes self-management educational programme. *Diabet Med* 2004; **21** (Suppl. 2): A84.

100. Byard AJ, Murphy HR, Skinner TC, Wadham CL, Rayman G. The development, evaluation and evolution of a paediatric carbohydrate counting programme from Families, Adolescents and Children Teamwork Study (FACTS). *Diabet Med* 2004; **21** (Suppl. 2): A86.

101. Anderson BJ. Diabetes self-care: lessons from research on the family and broader contexts. *Curr Diab Rep* 2003; **3** (2): 134–140.

102. Grey M, Boland EA, Davidson M, Yu C, Sullivan-Bolyai S, Tamborland WV. Short-term effects of coping skills training as adjunct to intensive therapy in adolescents. *Diabetes Care* 1998; **21** (6): 902–907.

103. Grey M, Boland EA, Davidson M, Li J, Tamborlane WV. Coping skills training for youth with diabetes mellitus has long-lasting effects on metabolic control and quality of life. *J Pediatr* 2000; **137** (1): 107–113.

104. Grey M, Berry D. Coping skills training and problem solving in diabetes. *Curr Diab Rep* 2004; **4** (2): 126–131.

105. Howells L, Wilson AC, Skinner TC, Newton R, Morris AD, Greene SA. A randomized control trial of the effect of negotiated telephone support on glycaemic control in young people with Type 1 diabetes. *Diabet Med* 2002; **19** (8): 643–648.
106. Channon S, Huws-Thomas MV, Gregory JW, Rollnick S. Motivational interviewing with teenagers with diabetes. *Clin Child Psychol Psychiatry* 2005; **10** (1): 43–51.
107. Miller WR, Rollnick S. *Motivational Interviewing: Preparing People to Change Addictive Behavior.* New York: Guilford, 1991.
108. Miller WR, Rollnick S. *Motivational Interviewing: Preparing People for Change* (2nd edn). New York: Guilford, 2002.
109. Dunn C, Deroo L, Rivara FP. The use of brief interventions adapted from motivational interviewing across behavioral domains: a systematic review. *Addiction* 2001; **96** (12): 1725–1742.
110. Burke BL, Arkowitz H, Menchola M. The efficacy of motivational interviewing: a meta-analysis of controlled clinical trials. *J Consult Clin Psychol* 2003; **71** (5): 843–861.
111. Lawendowski LA. A motivational intervention for adolescent smokers. *Prev Med* 1998; **27** (5 Pt 3): A39–A46.
112. Baer JS, Peterson PL. Motivational interviewing with adolescent and young adults. In Miller W, Rollnick S (eds), *Motivational Interviewing: Preparing People for Change.* New York: Guildford, 2002, pp 320–332.
113. Berg-Smith SM, Stevens VJ, Brown KM, Van Horn L, Gernhofer N, Peters E, Greenberg R, Snetselaar L, Ahrens L, Smith K. A brief motivational intervention to improve dietary adherence in adolescents. The Dietary Intervention Study in Children (DISC) Research Group. *Health Educ Res* 1999; **14** (3): 399–410.
114. Viner RM, Christie D, Taylor V, Hey S. Motivational/solution-focused intervention improves HbA1c in adolescents with Type 1 diabetes: a pilot study. *Diabet Med* 2004; **21** (s2): 111–120.
115. Rollnick S. Comments on Dunn et al.'s 'The use of brief interventions adapted from motivational interviewing across behavioral domains: a systematic review'. Enthusiasm, quick fixes and premature controlled trials. *Addiction* 2001; **96** (12): 1769–1770; discussion 1774–1775.
116. Heather N. Brief alcohol interventions have expanded in range but how they work is still mysterious. *Addiction* 2003; **98** (8): 1025–1026.
117. Huws-Thomas MV. *A Randomised Controlled Trial of Motivational Interviewing with Adolescents with Diabetes.* PhD Thesis. Cardiff: University of Wales College of Medicine, 2005.
118. Leventhal H, Nerenz DR, Steele DJ. Illness representation and coping with health threats. In Baum A, Taylor SE, Singer JE. (eds), *Handbook of Psychology and Health.* Killsdale, NJ: Erlbaum, 1984, pp 219–252.
119. Hampsom SE, Glasgow RE, Toobert DJ. Personal models of diabetes and their relations to self-care activities. *Health Psychol* 1990; **9** (5): 632–646.
120. Skinner TC, Hampson SE. Social support and personal models of diabetes in relation to self-care and well-being in adolescents with Type I diabetes mellitus. *J Adolescence* 1998; **21** (6): 703–715.
121. Skinner TC, Hampson SE, Fife-Schaw C. Personality, personal model beliefs, and self-care in adolescents and young adults with Type 1 diabetes. *Health Psychol* 2002; **21** (1): 61–70.
122. Lau RR, Bernard TM, Hartman KA. Further explorations of common-sense representations of common illnesses. *Health Psychol* 1989; **8** (2): 195–219.
123. Tamborlane WV, Bonfig W, Boland E. Recent advances in treatment of youth with Type 1 diabetes: better care through technology. *Diabet Med* 2001; **18** (11): 864–870.
124. Bandura A. Self-efficacy. *The Exercise of Control.* New York: Freeman, 1997.

125. Bagozzi RP, Edwards EA. Goal setting and goal pursuit in the regulation of body weight. *Psychol Health* 1998; **13** (4): 593–621.

126. Schwarzer R, Fuchs R. Changing risk behaviors and adopting health behaviors: the role of self-efficacy beliefs. In Bandura A (ed.), *Self-Efficacy in Changing Societies*. New York: Cambridge University Press, 1995, pp. 259–288.

127. Rollnick S, Mason P, Butler C. *Health Behavior Change: A Guide for Practitioners*. London: Churchill Livingstone, 1999.

128. Bandura A. The explanatory and predictive scope of self-efficacy theory. *J Soc Clin Psychol* 1986; **4** (3): 359–373.

129. Bandura A. Exercise of personal agency through the self-efficacy mechanism. In Schwarzer R (ed.), *Self-Efficacy: Thought Control of Action*. Washington, DC: Hemisphere, 1992, pp 3–38.

130. Ajzen I, Fishbein M. *Understanding the Attitudes and Predicting Social Behavior*. Englewood Cliffs, NJ: Prentice-Hall, 1980.

3
Psychological Issues in the Management of Diabetes and Pregnancy

Maurice G. A. J. Wouters and **Frank J. Snoek**

3.1   Introduction

Pregnancy has a significant impact on most women with diabetes mellitus. Diabetic women who become pregnant are faced with increasing demands in managing their diabetes as it responds to the pregnancy. In addition, they are subjected to intensified medical care focussed on possible foetal problems, such as birth defects and maldevelopment, and diabetes-related complications.

Diabetes mellitus in pregnancy is associated with an increased risk of pre-eclampsia, spontaneous abortions, foetal malformations, stillbirths, macrosomia and related neonatal morbidity. In the last decades, it has become clear that poor glycaemic control is an important determinant of these problems.[1,2] Achieving and maintaining optimum glucose regulation is considered of high relevance in minimizing the risk of these complications.

Unfortunately, diabetic women with good glycaemic control before and during pregnancy generally should not expect a normal rate of perinatal complications. In a prospective cohort study of 323 Dutch women with type 1 diabetes and overall good glycaemic control (HbA1c ≤ 7 per cent), it was noticed that the rates of congenital malformations, macrosomia and perinatal death were still increased 3.5- to 4.5-fold as compared with national data.[3]

Next and related to medical problems, important psychological issues may arise and need to be addressed as part of a multidisciplinary team approach.

Psychology in Diabetes Care   Edited by Frank J. Snoek and T. Chas Skinner

This chapter will highlight some of the psychological issues involved in diabetes care throughout different stages of pregnancy, from planning conception to delivery and beyond.

3.2   Prepregnancy

In general, maternal and perinatal complication rates are lower in diabetic women with lower HbA1c levels.[1-3] In this respect, it is considered important to counsel diabetic women who are planning to become pregnant about the reduction in complications that may be achieved by (further) improvement of glycaemic control.[4-6] Fertile women with diabetes should be strongly encouraged to use effective contraception until optimal glycaemic control has been established.

Research suggests that most women with diabetes tend to seek medical care *after* they have discovered they are pregnant. In the Maine study, in which health care providers in a state-wide network were trained in preconception care and attempts were made to contact diabetic women before pregnancy, only one-third of the diabetic pregnancies occurred in women who had received preconception counselling.[7]

Lower income, unemployment, less education and unmarried status are known factors to have a major impact on whether or not women seek preconception care.[8]

Large individual differences may be observed in how diabetic women and their partners cope with the need for 'preconception watchfulness' and pregnancy planning. While some women or couples may be 'unrealistically' optimistic regarding the health risks involved, others may react over-anxiously, and develop a phobia of hyperglycaemia, leading to excessive blood glucose monitoring and very frequent consultations of the diabetes health care team.

Unplanned pregnancy may cause emotional stress and fears of criticism.

In a recent study, it was found that women who felt their doctor discouraged pregnancy were more likely to have an unplanned pregnancy than women who had been reassured they could have a healthy baby.[9] This finding underscores the importance of the doctor–patient relationship.[10]

Social support appears to play a significant role as well. In the same study, women with unplanned pregnancies reported to be less satisfied with their partner relationship than those who planned their pregnancies. Most of the women with unplanned pregnancies felt that their partners were not well informed about the possible risks or were not able to understand the amount of effort required to achieve a good diabetes control.[9]

3.3   Pregnancy

For a woman with diabetes the 'developmental tasks' related to pregnancy are essentially the same as for any woman, i.e. developing attachment to the foetus, preparing for separation and adopting a realistic relationship with the new-born.[11,12]

It is thought, however, that women with diabetes have a different mood profile compared with non-diabetic women. In a study of pregnant women with pre-existing diabetes mellitus and non-diabetic controls, maternal characteristics and test results on the Profile of Mood States—Bipolar form were reported. Women with diabetes displayed a greater anxiety and hostility in comparison with non-diabetic women with no association to their level of glycaemic control. Their psychological profile was not associated with the severity of the disease as reflected by the diabetes classification.[13]

By contrast, in a prospective longitudinal study using Mental Health Inventory (MHI-5) forms and the Spielberger State–Trait Anxiety Inventory (STAI) during pregnancy, women with gestational diabetes expressed no higher anxiety scores than glucose-tolerant women.[14] In a study measuring bipolar subjective mood states, the mood profile in such women was significantly associated with their level of glycaemic control.[15] Thus the degree of metabolic control appears of psychological importance in women with gestational diabetes. Continuous reassurance regarding metabolic control in women with gestational diabetes may enhance their confidence and ability to cope with their temporary disease state.[16]

The experience of pregnancy for a woman with diabetes is strongly influenced by the increasing demands of the diabetes treatment regimen, concerns about the health of her baby, and the impact of the pregnancy on her own health.

For women who are in poor metabolic control, the requirements of more intensive self-care and medical management can give way to worries and increased stress levels.

Women striving for 'perfect' diabetes control may find it extremely difficult to accept any elevated blood glucose level and become highly frustrated by the day-to-day glucose variability that is likely to occur in insulin-dependent diabetes regardless of pregnancy. Lowering of glycosylated haemoglobin can help to decrease stress levels and improve self-esteem. Failure to improve glycaemic control can easily lead to feelings of guilt and an increase of psychological distress and eventually diabetes 'burn-out'.[17]

Strict glycaemic control increases the risk of (severe) hypoglycaemia. It was found that in about two-thirds of diabetic pregnancies that were regulated by intensive insulin therapy, at least one episode of severe hypoglycaemia occurred during the first 20 weeks.[18] In a recent cohort-study, a mean of 2.6 episodes of hypoglycaemia was reported during the first trimester. A lower HbA1c level and a higher total daily insulin dose were predictive for severe hypoglycaemia.[19]

Severe hypoglycaemia can cause high levels of anxiety, confronting the mother-to-be with a serious dilemma. On the one hand she strives for optimal glycaemic control to reduce the risk of birth defects; on the other hand she wants to minimize the risk of hypoglycaemia because of the possible harm that it may cause to herself and the foetus. To date, the adverse effects of (periods of) maternal hypoglycaemia to the foetus's health are not well established.

Impaired hypoglycaemia awareness and related worries about severe hypoglycaemia can lead the pregnant woman to accept higher levels of blood glucose, thereby compromising glycaemic control.[20] This may be particularly true for women for whom work and/or family commitments make it extremely difficult to have low blood glucose levels.

Obstetrical care in the first and early second trimesters is largely concentrated on detecting birth defects. In the late second and third trimester, the obstetrical focus is on assessing foetal growth and development, and maternal health.

The revelation of foetal anomalies, abnormal foetal growth and/or development in women with poor metabolic control may cause feelings of guilt and distress, resulting in further glucose dysregulation.

Clinical studies suggest a higher occurrence of premature labour and preterm delivery in diabetic pregnancies.[21,22] The imminent birth of a preterm infant and a (long) period of hospital stay preceding this event may induce anxiety and feelings of separation in women concerned. This emotional stress can have a negative impact on their metabolic control and vice versa.

3.4 Delivery

Delivery is a stressful event to all women and their partners. In general, women are in fear of the possible pain that delivery may cause. Women may be anxious whether they will be able to cope with this pain if analgesia is not available soon or is not effective enough. In women with diabetes, stress levels may be increased in view of the possible complications of delivery related to macrosomia. Shoulder dystocia due to macrosomia is a major clinical problem which may cause irreversible physical damage to the newborn and secondary surgical complications to the mother. Feelings of anger, doubt and anxiety may persist for many years thereafter. In this respect, it is important to discuss prenatally the procedures and possible complications of either vaginal or caesarean delivery.

3.5 Lactation

Little is known about the psychological implications of breastfeeding in women with diabetes other than in non-diabetic women. Diabetic women may find it stimulating that breastfeeding appears to be an independent protective factor against type 1 diabetes in their children.[23]

3.6 Childhood

Little is known about how diabetic pregnancy, both in type 1 and gestational diabetes, affects the development of the maternal–infant relationship. There is some research to suggest that children from diabetic mothers are at increased risk for a variety of behavioural disturbances, partly related to the children's obesity.[24]

In an Israeli study, one-year-old infants of women with diabetes mellitus had lower scores on the Bayley Scales of Infant Development and revealed fewer positive and more negative behaviours than infants of mothers in the non-diabetic group. Infant outcomes in the maternal diabetic group were associated with maternal metabolism.[25]

3.7 Practice Implications

Prepregnancy counselling has so far shown to have a limited effect in changing contraceptive behaviour in women with diabetes. Unplanned pregnancies therefore remain a major problem. Further research into possible ways of improving the efficacy of prepregnancy programmes are warranted. Such studies should take into account socio-economic, cultural and ethnic factors, that can strongly influence a woman's acceptance, understanding and adherence to restrictions imposed by a diabetic pregnancy.[26]

Education is a prequisite for adequate diabetes self-management, but by no means a guarantee that patients will indeed adhere to the diabetes regimen. In order to help women to cope more effectively with their diabetes, it is essential to identify their specific psychological and behavioural barriers, such as low diabetes self-efficacy, fear of hypoglycaemia and lack of social support. Customized psychosocial interventions should prove helpful in improving the outcome of diabetic pregnancies as well as the women's quality of life.

New technologies in monitoring glycaemic control should be evaluated regarding their psychological implications. Continuous glucose monitoring (CGM) is a promising technique that appears useful in detecting high postprandial blood glucose levels and nocturnal hypoglycaemic events that are unrecognized by intermittent blood glucose measurements.[27] The psychological consequences of CGM in pregnant diabetic women who are confronted with concealed high and low levels of blood glucose despite tight monitoring should be a subject of future studies.

The importance of a follow-up protocol after delivery is emphasized by the observation that glycaemic control often quickly deteriorates after delivery, returning to suboptimal prepregnancy levels.

In the last decades, much progress has been made in the medical management of diabetic pregnancy. A large number of health care professionals is involved in the medical care for pregnant women with diabetes. Dedicated medical specialists (obstetricians, endocrinologists, opthalmologists, nephrologists, neonatologists), diabetic nurses and dietary consultants have their specific shares in the prevention, diagnosis and treatment of maternal and perinatal complications. In daily practice, it appears difficult to attune the activities of these different professionals to each other. In Amsterdam (VU medical center), an integrated pregnancy and diabetes clinic was started in April 2004 to overcome these problems and improve the care for the pregnant woman with diabetes and her child (-to-be). The rates of complications and women's satisfaction with the provided care will be evaluated and used to further improve the quality of care.

Next to the medical aspects of diabetic pregnancy, psychological and social issues appear to be important determinants of pregnancy outcome and possibly provide a key to further enhancement of diabetes care in pregnancy. The integration of psychological expertise with specialized medical care may provide a substantial contribution to a further improvement of multidisciplinary diabetes management in pregnancy.

References

1. Miller E, Hare JW, Cloherty JP *et al*. Elevated maternal haemoglobin A1c in early pregnancy and major congenital anomalies in infants of diabetic mothers. *N Engl J Med* 1981; **304**: 1331–1334.
2. Diabetes Control and Complications Trial (DCCT) Research Group. Pregnancy outcomes in the Diabetes Control and Complications Trial. *Am J Obstet Gynecol* 1996; **174**: 1343–1353.
3. Evers IM, De Valk HW, Visser GHA. Risk of complications of pregnancy in women with type 1 diabetes: nationwide prospective study in the Netherlands. *BMJ* 2004; **328**: 915–919.
4. Kitzmiller JL, Gavin LA, Gin GD *et al*. Preconception care of diabetes: glycemic control prevents congenital anomalies. *JAMA* 1991; **265**: 731–736.
5. Ray JG, O'Brien TE, Chan WS. Preconception care and the risk of congenital anomalies in the offspring of women with diabetes mellitus: a meta-analysis. *Q J Med* 2001; **4**: 435–444.
6. American Diabetes Association. Preconception care of women with diabetes. Position Statement. *Diabetes Care* 2004; **27**: s76–s78.
7. Wilhoite MB, Bennert HW Jr, Palomaki GE *et al*. The impact of preconception counseling on pregnancy outcomes. The experience of the Maine pregnancy program. *Diabetes Care* 1993; **16**: 450–455.
8. Janz NK, Herman WH, Becker MP *et al*. Diabetes and pregnancy: factors associated with seeking pre-conception care. *Diabetes Care* 1995; **18**: 157–165.
9. Holing EV, Beyer CS, Brown ZA, Connell FA. Why don't women with diabetes plan their pregnancies? *Diabetes Care* 1998; **21**: 889–895.
10. Coustan DR. Pre-conception planning. The relationship's the thing (Editorial). *Diabetes Care* 1998; **21**: 887–888.
11. Caplan G. Emotional implications of pregnancy, and influences on family relationships. In Stuart HC, Prugh DG (eds), *The Healthy Child*. Cambridge: Harvard University Press, 1960, pp 72–81.
12. Kay E. Psychosocial responses to pregnant women with diabetes. In Brown FM, Hare JW (eds), *Diabetes Complicating Pregnancy: the Joslin Clinic Method*. London: Wiley, 1995, pp 199–213.

13. Langer N, Langer O. Pre-existing diabetics: relationship between glycemic control and emotional status in pregnancy. *J Matern Fetal Med* 1998; **7**: 257–263.
14. Daniells S, Grenyer BF, Davis WS, Coleman KJ, Burgess JA, Moses RG. Gestational diabetes mellitus; is a diagnosis associated with increase in maternal anxiety and stress in the short and intermediate term? *Diabetes Care* 2003; **26**: 385–389.
15. Langer N, Langer O. Comparison of pregnancy mood profiles in gestational diabetes and preexisting diabetes. *Diabetes Educ* 2000; **26**: 667–672.
16. Langer N, Langer O. Emotional adjustment to diagnosis and intensified treatment of gestational diabetes. *Obstet Gynecol* 1994; **84**: 329–334.
17. Polonsky WH. Understanding and treating patients with diabetes burnout. In Anderson BJ, Rubin RR (eds), *Practical Psychology for Diabetes Clinicians*. Alendria: ADA, 1996, pp 183–192.
18. Rosenn BM, Miodovnik M, Holcberg G, Khoury JC, Siddiqi TA. Hypoglycemia: the price of intensive insulin therapy for pregnant women with insulin-dependent diabetes mellitus. *Obstet Gynecol* 1995; **85**: 417–422.
19. Evers IM, Ter Braak EWMT, De Valk HW, Van der Schoot B, Janssen N, Visser GHA. Risk indicators predictive for severe hypoglycemia during the first trimester of type 1 diabetes pregnancy. *Diabetes Care* 2002; **25**: 554–559.
20. Kimmerle R, Heinemann L, Delecki A, Berger M. Severe hypoglycemia incidence and predisposing factors in 85 pregnancies of type 1 diabetic women. *Diabetes Care* 1992; **15**: 1034–1037.
21. Sibai BM, Caritis SN, Hauth JC *et al*. Preterm delivery in women with pregestational diabetes mellitus or chronic hypertension relative to women with uncomplicated pregnancies. *Am J Obstet Gynecol* 2000; **183**: 1520–1524.
22. Hedderson MM, Ferrara A, Sacks DA. Gestational diabetes mellitus and lesser degrees of pregnancy hyperglycemia: association with increased risk of spontaneous preterm birth. *Obstet Gynecol* 2003; **102**: 850–856.
23. Sadauskaité-Kuehne V, Ludvigsson J, Padaiga Z, Jašinskiené E, Samuelsson U. Longer breastfeeding is an independent protective factor against development of type 1 diabetes mellitus in childhood. *Diabetes Metab Res Rev* 2004; **20**: 150–157.
24. Rizzo TA, Silverman BL, Metzger BE, Cho NH. Behavioral adjustment in children of diabetic mothers. *Acta Paed* 1997; **86**: 969–974.
25. Levy-Shiff R, Lerman M, Har-Even D, Hod M. Maternal adjustment and infant outcome in medically defined high risk pregnancy. *Dev Psychol* 2002; **38**: 93–103.
26. Wootton J, Girling JC. Addressing the needs of the inner city clinics. In Dornhorst A, Hadden DR (eds), *Diabetes and Pregnancy. An International Approach to Diagnosis and Management*. Chichester: Wiley, 1996, pp 265–276.
27. Yogev Y, Chen R, Ben-Haroush A, Phillip M, Jovanovic L, Hod M. Continuous glucose monitoring for the evaluation of gravid women with type 1 diabetes mellitus. *Obstet Gynecol* 2003; **101**: 633–638.

4

Diabetes in Older Adults

Marie Clark and **Koula G. Asimakopoulou**

4.1   Introduction

Diabetes mellitus is a common metabolic disorder affecting older adults. With time, effects of diabetes on the cardiovascular system, the kidneys, the retina and the peripheral nervous system, often referred to as long-term complications of diabetes, substantially increase mortality and morbidity in older adults. In general, diabetes in older adults is underdiagnosed and undertreated. A growing body of evidence assessing outcomes of interventions and an increasing number of therapeutic options for diabetes management have increased the importance of making a diagnosis and offering appropriate intervention strategies to older persons who have this potentially devastating disorder. Although the incidence of new-onset type 1 diabetes in older adults is very low, effective treatment of type 1 diabetes may prevent or delay the development of long-term complications and increased mortality. Thus, people who develop type 1 diabetes earlier in life may live to old age and therefore become a part of the spectrum of diabetes mellitus in an older adult population.

Approximately 90 per cent of older adults with diabetes have type 2 diabetes. Worldwide, type 2 diabetes is an important and common disease that is steadily becoming more common. In Europe, the USA and most westernized countries, type 2 accounts for up to 85 per cent of total cases of diabetes, and probably affects five to seven per cent of the population; it is likely that many cases (perhaps up to 50 per cent) are currently undiagnosed.[1,2]

The prevalence of type 2 diabetes is low (less than one per cent) in many developing societies and very high (40–50 per cent) in certain groups, e.g. the Pima Indians of Arizona and the Nauruans.[2,3] Both of these societies have become westernized relatively rapidly during the last few decades, and this has been

Psychology in Diabetes Care   Edited by Frank J. Snoek and T. Chas Skinner
© 2005 John Wiley & Sons, Ltd.

paralleled by an increase in the incidence of type 2 diabetes. Several key aspects of the westernized lifestyle ('coca-colonization'[3]) predispose to obesity, insulin resistance and type 2 diabetes, notably a high intake of energy-rich fatty foods and physical inactivity. The diabetogenic effects of westernization are also illustrated by the several-fold increases in the prevalence of type 2 diabetes seen in immigrant populations, such as Asians living in the UK or South Africa.[3,4]

Type 2 diabetes is predominantly, but not exclusively, a disease of the middle-aged and elderly. In Europe and the USA, about 70 per cent of patients are over 55 years of age and the average age at diagnosis is 60 years. The prevalence of type 2 diabetes increases markedly with age in all populations, and in Europe and the USA it probably affects 10 per cent or more of those over 70 years of age. The true prevalence is difficult to judge because many cases have few or no symptoms in the early stages, and are therefore undiagnosed.[5,6] Overall, there appears to be a male preponderance (approximately 3:2 males:females).

Type 2 diabetes is a very costly disease, in individual, social and economic terms. Although sometimes asymptomatic, it can cause the same microvascular and macrovascular complications as type 1. Accelerated and severe atherosclerosis is the major problem and results in much morbidity through angina, heart failure, claudication and stroke; myocardial infarction, often at a young age, is the most common cause of death in type 2 diabetes. Retinopathy, nephropathy and neuropathy can all affect patients with type 2 diabetes. It cannot therefore be regarded as 'mild' diabetes, even though blood glucose levels may be only moderately raised in many cases and patients will not die acutely if treatment is withdrawn.[7]

Institutionalized older adults with diabetes

Since diabetes is one of the commonest chronic diseases of older adults, one might expect a higher prevalence of diabetes and its complications in residential or nursing homes. Several US studies have found diabetes in 20 per cent of nursing home residents[8] and in one study almost 90 per cent of diabetic residents had coronary artery disease, strokes or peripheral vascular disease, with 6.4 major diagnoses compared with only 2.4 in non-diabetic residents. In the UK, Sinclair et al.[9] report an overall prevalence rate of 12 per cent for known diabetes, and 14.8 per cent for newly detected diabetes in care home residents. Looking at the patterns of care, levels of complications and resource usage of diabetic residents in residential or nursing homes in the UK, Benbow et al.[10] surveyed 44 residential and nursing homes comparing residents with diabetes with age- and sex-matched controls. The provision of care for this vulnerable group of diabetic residents was found to be inadequate despite their high morbidity levels and greater use of health service resources. Many residents had no medical team responsible for their diabetic care and had not been assessed for the presence or risk of diabetic complications, emphasizing that diabetes care in institutionalized older adults is potentially a long neglected area.

4.2 The Ageing Process

There are currently over 57 million people resident in the UK. The relative proportion of elderly people (aged 65 years or over) in this population has increased considerably and the proportion aged over 80 years shows an even more dramatic rise. In the UK in 1971, 10.9 per cent of the population were aged between 65 and 79 with 2.3 per cent over 80. The number of people over pensionable age is projected to increase from 11.2 million in 2006 to 11.9 million in 2011, and will rise to 13.1 million by 2021[11] (Table 3.2). These trends are also reflected in other European countries. In the USA, 12.6 per cent of the population were aged 65 or over in 1990. This proportion is expected to rise to 22.9 per cent by the year 2050 with the over 85 year old group increasing by a factor of 3.9 in this timescale.[12]

Ageing has been defined '... as a process that converts healthy adults into frail ones, with diminished reserves in most physiological systems and an exponentially increasing vulnerability to most diseases and death'.[13] It is difficult to distinguish between what constitutes natural ageing and what constitutes accelerated ageing due to disease processes among elderly patients. Cross-sectional studies, comparing findings in elderly people with those in younger people, have helped to highlight changes associated with the ageing process. In certain organs, such as the kidneys, a subgroup of people appear to experience a gradual decline in function over time, roughly a one per cent loss in function per year starting around the age of 30, while in others function remains constant well into old age.[12] Such changes will obviously have a profound effect on drugs which are dependent on the kidney for elimination. Age-related changes in the eye including decreased pupil size and growth of the lens lead to decreased accommodation, acuity, colour sensitivity and depth of perception,[12] which can lead to difficulties for older people in distinguishing between tablets that look similar.

It is important to note that ageing is a gradual process, with many changes commencing in early adulthood, although most do not manifest themselves until later life. In addition, not everyone ages at the same rate or in the same way. Frequently, the process of ageing only becomes apparent when a particular organ is subjected to external stress; for example, older people may often have a normal resting pulse but cannot sufficiently increase cardiac output to cope with exercise.

There is considerable debate about whether the age-related decline in insulin action, for example, is an effect of age per se or is secondary to age-related changes in body composition and physical activity. An absolute or relative increase of body adiposity, particularly central body adiposity, and an associated decrease of muscle mass can each contribute to insulin resistance. Similarly, it is well known that conditions associated with decreased physical activity are associated with insulin resistance and that exercise training can improve insulin sensitivity. Thus, diminished physical activity in an older individual can also contribute to decreased insulin sensitivity. Both in animal studies and in humans, it has been difficult to demonstrate a residual effect of ageing on insulin action when the changes in body composition and physical activity are controlled for.

Coexisting illness can be another confounding factor affecting insulin sensitivity in an older person. Furthermore, any acute illness can precipitate hyperglycaemia because of effects of stress hormones released during stressful illness to inhibit insulin secretion.

Ageing is further associated with a myth of gradual yet inescapable cognitive decline. It is well established that impairments in cognitive functioning are often seen with advancing age but that such a decline is not an 'all or none' phenomenon. That is, age does not seem to affect all areas of cognition and all older adults in the same way.[14] For example, it is generally accepted that over-learned, well practised, familiar cognitive skills (i.e. ones relying on crystallized intelligence) are likely to be spared, whereas activities requiring reasoning and complex problem solving (i.e. fluid intelligence) may well be affected by the ageing process.[15]

4.3 Symptoms and their Representation

Because the symptoms of diabetes in older adults are often slow to develop, less severe and longer lasting, and because they appear against a more complex background of somatic sensations, older persons may have difficulty distinguishing illness specific symptoms from those attributed to normal ageing, creating unnecessary risk for morbidity and mortality. Indeed, Kart[16] has suggested that physicians, as well as older adults themselves, overestimate the changes that are caused by biological ageing, physicians often assuming that physical and intellectual debilitation necessarily come with age and should be expected as a consequence of ageing. One consequence of older adults' acceptance of symptoms as signs of ageing is that they fail to report these symptoms to health care professionals.[17] This type of misattribution could be important if it leads to the discounting and ignoring of diabetes symptoms or of delay in diagnosis and treatment.[18]

Experimental evidence of the existence of an age–illness rule was reported by Prohaska et al.[19] They presented participants with scenarios depicting symptoms of varying severity and duration and found that the likelihood of attributing symptoms to ageing was greater for mild than severe symptoms. Attributions of symptoms to age rather than illness also occurred more frequently for older than younger participants regardless of the severity and duration of the symptoms. Participants who attributed symptoms to age also reported less emotional distress and more delay in care-seeking than participants who attributed symptoms to illness – this held for participants of all ages. The data was also clear in showing that all patients were more likely to delay care-seeking when they initially attributed symptoms to ageing.

Extrapolation from these data suggests that older individuals with diabetes may be at greater risk because they are somewhat more likely to make ageing attributions and, because older persons are less robust and resistant to pathogens, they may suffer more if they do delay in seeking care for their illness. Thus, while stimuli, such as gradual onset of symptoms, that lead to ageing attributions and their behavioural consequences are similar for younger and older persons,[20] negative health consequences of errors induced by such attributions are more likely for the older individual with diabetes.

In contrast to these findings, however, it is of interest to note that work with people with type 2 diabetes has shown that they are more likely than healthy controls to report a greater frequency and severity of memory problems, which do not appear to be supported by objective memory testing.[21] This subjective, yet apparently erroneous, symptom reporting is potentially worrying in that it has also been associated with poorer diabetes-specific problem solving in type 2 patients.[22] Clinicians may hence benefit from the knowledge that their elderly patients with type 2 diabetes may over-emphasize memory problems, which, although not objectively evident, may well moderate attempts to self-manage successfully.

4.4 Clinical Features of Diabetes

The clinical picture of type 2 diabetes differs from that of type 1 in several important aspects. The older age of onset of most patients has already been mentioned. Just over 50 per cent of cases present with classical hyperglycaemic symptoms, but with rare exceptions (e.g. during intercurrent illness) the features of diabetic ketoacidosis are absent. Many type 2 patients do not complain of obvious diabetic symptoms, and the disease is detected either opportunistically, for example by screening at medical examinations or during hospital visits, or when patients present with intercurrent infections, usually genital candidiasis (particularly in women) or of the urinary tract or skin. Some present with complications of diabetes itself, such as myocardial infarction or peripheral vascular disease, or with microvascular disease, most commonly retinopathy, which may be discovered by an optician during a routine eye test. The high proportion of incidental diagnoses in apparently asymptomatic people emphasizes the fact that type 2 diabetes runs an insidious course; various studies have estimated that significant hyperglycaemia is present on average for 5–7 years before the diagnosis is made. These data also indicate that many patients with overt type 2 diabetes still remain undiagnosed, and several surveys that have systematically screened defined populations suggest that up to 50 per cent of all cases have not yet been detected.[23]

4.5   Diabetes Complications in Older Adults

Chronic complications

Older adults with diabetes are susceptible to all the usual complications of diabetes. Although clinical outcomes of many of the diabetes complications including end-stage renal disease, loss of vision, myocardial infarction, stroke, peripheral vascular disease, and peripheral neuropathy all increase with age in the absence of diabetes, their incidence and co-occurrence are all exaggerated by the presence of diabetes. Indeed, there is substantial evidence that the presence of diabetes in an older adult increases risk for adverse outcomes.

Overall, it is estimated that a diagnosis of diabetes is associated on average with a 10-year reduction in life expectancy. However, this figure becomes progressively reduced at advanced old age, when risks of competing causes of mortality rise exponentially. Nonetheless, diabetes is associated with a higher mortality rate at any age, approaching twice the rate in older people of comparable age without diabetes in some studies. Similarly, the rates of myocardial infarction, stroke, and end-stage renal disease are increased approximately twofold, and the risk of visual loss is increased by approximately 40 per cent in older people with diabetes. This level of increased relative risk may appear modest on an individual level. However, since the elderly population has by far the highest rates of these conditions, the increase in absolute risk is more substantial. Thus a twofold relative risk increase represents a very large number of added adverse outcomes. The risk for lower extremity amputation is dramatically increased in older people with diabetes, approximately 10-fold greater than that for older people without diabetes.

Macrovascular complications

The individual with type 2 diabetes is more likely to be affected by arterial disease, partly because type 2 diabetes generally appears at a time of life when arteriosclerotic problems are frequent even in the non-diabetic population. In addition, these patients frequently have many other adverse arteriosclerotic risk factors such as obesity, hyperlipidaemia, hypertension (which is more common in diabetic people[24]) and smoking. The grouping of these risk factors has long been recognized and has been given the title of 'syndrome X' by Reaven,[25] who has suggested that insulin resistance in various tissues can explain its key features.

Obesity is a major predisposing factor to insulin resistance and is also an important obstacle to the effective management of type 2 diabetes. In the UK and other westernized countries, at least 50 per cent of men and 70 per cent of women are 120 per cent of the ideal body weight at presentation;[26] truncal obesity, which is associated with hypertension, dyslipidaemia and cardiovascular disease is particularly common.[27]

Coronary artery disease is the main complication of type 2 diabetes. Angina affects 17 per cent or more of patients[7] and ultimately nearly 60 per cent die from ischaemic heart disease as compared with 15 per cent of patients with type 1 diabetes.[28] Myocardial infarction is more common in diabetes and also carries a worse prognosis;[29,30] the mortality rate is about twice that in non-diabetic individuals. Peripheral vascular disease may cause intermittent claudication and gangrene of the foot or leg, sometimes requiring amputation. Together with neuropathy, it is a major cause of diabetic foot syndrome, a source of considerable morbidity and cost to the health services. Cerebrovascular disease presents as transient ischaemic attacks or stroke, which is more common amongst diabetic patients and carries a higher mortality than in the non-diabetic population.[28,29]

Microvascular complications

The specific microvascular complications of diabetes may be less prominent in type 2 diabetes than in type 1 but they still provide cause for concern. Retinopathy and cataracts each affect about 15 per cent of patients and may result in a significant loss of independence for these individuals. Maculopathy is an especially common form of retinopathy in type 2 and may threaten vision;[31] it may be very difficult to diagnose at routine fundoscopy. By contrast, proliferative retinopathy, the most common cause of blindness in type 1 diabetes, is rare. Nephropathy is probably as likely to develop in type 2 as it is in type 1, although its prevalence is lower because most type 2 patients, being substantially older, have a shorter exposure to hyperglycaemia and therefore less opportunity to progress to end-stage nephropathy with renal failure. In addition, because type 2 diabetes is now so common, these patients constitute the majority of those requiring renal replacement therapy in many countries. Finally, neuropathy is a common complication and causes serious morbidity in a substantial proportion of type 2 patients, about eight per cent of whom have painful, rather than asymptomatic, neuropathy.[7] At least one-third of male type 2 patients, when directly questioned, have some degree of erectile dysfunction.[32]

Psychological complications

Cognitive decline

Research on cognitive function in older people with type 2 diabetes has been performed primarily by small, cross-sectional studies and, to a lesser extent, by epidemiological studies involving much larger samples. Within each type of study, however, the evidence generated has been inconsistent. There are two main reasons for this lack of consensus. First, older people with diabetes usually also have other medical conditions that impair cognitive functioning, such as hypertension and cardiovascular disease. Therefore, identifying the independent contributions of diabetes and of other conditions, or indeed controlling for the influence of the latter, presents a challenge for researchers.[33,34] Second, there is a lack of consensus over the cognitive functions that ought to be tested, as well as the assessment instruments that should be used. As a result, no two studies have used the identical test battery.

Factors that may further complicate the relationship between cognitive function and diabetes are age, duration of illness, diabetes complications and glycaemic control and these have been considered in research studies in the field. However, separating the unique contribution of these factors is a challenge that has yet to be met.

Notwithstanding these difficulties, simple and more complex cognitive processes have been studied. In general, performance on complex cognitive tasks such as those assessing abstract reasoning, verbal memory and mental flexibility has often been shown to be impaired in people with type 2 diabetes.[35–37] Learning and memory in particular have further been proposed to be affected by older age.[38] More complicated diabetes[39] and a longer illness duration[40] are also related to greater cognitive decline in patients with the illness.

Finally, a recent review of prospective studies[41] has also concluded that type 2 diabetes may well be associated with a higher probability of cognitive decline or indeed accelerated dementia. The strength of prospective studies lies in the fact that they have examined large samples, and hence are powerful enough to detect small changes in cognitive performance; however, at the same time, they suffer from methodological difficulties such as relying on patient self-report for diagnosis of the illness,[40] failing to control for pre-morbid intelligence[42] or using crude measures of dementia (the Mini Mental State Examination, MMSE).[43]

We conclude that older people with type 2 diabetes are more likely to have some cognitive impairment in comparison to people without the illness. However, such impairment is probably limited to relatively complex cognitive processes and may be attributable to other conditions that often accompany diabetes and that are likely to interfere with cognitive function. The precise extent and severity of cognitive impairment is unlikely to be established until a consensus is achieved on the cognitive functions that should be routinely assessed and on the precise battery of cognitive tests that is likely to be sensitive enough to detect these cognitive changes.

So what are the implications of these findings for the management of older adults with diabetes? Although much research has been conducted to investigate the extent and magnitude of diabetes-related deterioration in cognitive performance, few studies have attempted to relate these findings to diabetes self-management. In other words, although most researchers in the field warn of potential cognitive decline in patients with the illness, only very few[44,22] have explored the extent to which cognitive function predicts diabetes self-management in patients with type 2 diabetes. From the limited amount of work in this area it would appear that cognitive performance is *not* a major predictor of diabetes self-care activities in older adults with the illness. In our work[22] we found only moderate relationships between performance on a battery of cognitive tests and diabetes self-care as assessed by self-report, suggesting that the relatively small changes in cognitive function that we observed may not be a severe threat to self-management of the illness. Interestingly, we also found that patients' subjective perceptions of their everyday memory performance, rather than objective neuro-psychological test performance, is associated with diabetes-related problem solving activities in older people with the illness. These findings would suggest that clinicians should be aware that some of their type 2 patients may well be suffering from cognitive difficulties, over and above those that would be expected as a result of old age and other commorbidities. This cognitive decline, however, is unlikely to heavily compromise self-care efforts; instead, patients' beliefs about their cognitive function may well be more useful in predicting diabetes self-management.

Depression and anxiety

Older people are well known to be less depressed and less anxious than their younger counterparts.[45] Chronically ill older patients are also less likely than their younger chronically ill counterparts to be depressed or anxious.[46] Diabetes, however, has been extensively reported to be associated with both depressive illness and anxiety disorder. Although depression is not particularly more prevalent in diabetes than the rates reported in other chronic illnesses,[47] it is more prevalent among people with diabetes than the general population, affecting around 15–20 per cent of patients. Women with type 2 diabetes are twice as likely as men to be depressed,[48] with body weight a significant predictor of depressive illness. Diabetes complications such as neuropathy, retinopathy, macrovascular complications and sexual dysfunction have also been associated with depressive illness;[49] however, the presence of uncomplicated diabetes in the absence of another chronic illness does not seem to predispose to depression.[50]

The aetiology of depression in older adults with diabetes is not yet clear, although both physiological and psychological factors have been explored.[51] Recent work[52] has indicated that depression increases diabetes symptoms by complicating patients' self-care efforts. In particular, it has been proposed[53] that depression affects diabetes self-management in three distinctive ways: first by affecting older patients' overall quality of life,[54] second by reducing physical activity levels (which have been shown to be restored with depression treatment[55]) and third by impairing patients' ability to communicate effectively with their heath care teams.

Depression in diabetes remains underdiagnosed and undertreated. The few studies that have been conducted to investigate treatment effectiveness have produced encouraging results. Lustman et al.[56] showed that cognitive behavioral therapy (CBT) was effective in remitting depression, although these results were compromised in the presence of diabetes complications and lower frequency of blood glucose testing. In similar work,[56] CBT was found to be effective in reducing glycosylated haemoglobin 6 months after treatment. In more recent work, Williams and his team[55] showed that a combined care approach for depression improved diabetes patients' depressive symptoms and their overall functioning as well as their weekly frequency of physical activity. HbA1c levels were unaffected.

Overall, and as Snoek and Skinner[51] (p. 265) have argued, '...evidence to support the effect of psychological treatment in problematic diabetes is still scarce...'. This is not just true for depression, but also for anxiety disorder. A review of anxiety prevalence rates in diabetes patients[57] showed that around 14 per cent of patients have clinical characteristics of generalized anxiety disorder (GAD), whilst around 40 per cent present with elevated symptoms of anxiety, with the presence of elevated symptoms being significantly higher in women (around 55 per cent) than men.

At the moment, routine depression and anxiety screening and treatment are not processes that are a routine part of diabetes care in general. Given the high prevalence of both disorders however, and their potentially devastating effect on diabetes self-care, routine screening of the older patient with diabetes is recommended.

Physical disability

Diabetes is also associated with greater risks of disabilities related to mobility and daily tasks among older adults.[58,59] Findings from the National Health and Nutrition and Examination Surveys indicate that people with diabetes have about two to three times the prevalence of inability to walk 400 metres, do housework, prepare meals and manage money. One-quarter of diabetic women 60 years of age and older report being unable to walk 400 metres, compared with less than one-sixth of non-diabetic women of the same age. Diabetic women become disabled at approximately twice the rate of non-diabetic women and have an increased risk of falls and hip fractures.[59,60]

The association of diabetes with physical disability is explained in part by classic complications of diabetes (for example, coronary heart disease and visual impairment), but a 60 per cent excess prevalence of disability remains after controlling for these factors. The mechanisms explaining the association are probably multifactorial. In NHANES III, CHD and high body mass index (BMI) were the strongest explanatory factors among women, accounting for 52 per cent of their excess risk for disability.[58] Among men, CHD and stroke were the most important explanatory factors, explaining 25 and 21 per cent of the excess disability risk, respectively. These findings were supported in a number of further studies.[59,61] In all of these studies, however, a significant excess risk of disability associated with diabetes remained, even after controlling for diabetes-related complications. This indicates either that diabetes has an intrinsic influence on disability or that other unmeasured or undiscovered diabetes-related complications influence the risk for disability.

4.6 Mortality in Type 2 Diabetes

Five-year mortality in type 2 diabetes is increased two-to-threefold, and age-adjusted life expectancy is reduced by 5–10 years compared with the general population.[62,63] Interestingly, the mortality risk does not seem particularly related to the duration of the disease;[64] indeed, for type 2 patients diagnosed over the age of 75 years, mortality is similar to that of their age-matched, non-diabetic counterparts.[65]

4.7 Diabetes Control and Complications

The natural history of microvascular and neuropathic complications in type 2 diabetes has been difficult to define because the disease may be present for many years before it is diagnosed, and the incidence and progression of complications may be influenced by multiple confounding factors including age and hypertension. Nevertheless, hyperglycaemia is clearly associated with the presence and progression of microvascular complications in type 2 diabetes.[66–68]

The recently reported UK Prospective Diabetes Study (UKPDS), a multicentre, prospective, randomized clinical trial, was designed to determine whether improved blood glucose control would prevent complications and reduce morbidity and mortality in patients with newly diagnosed type 2 diabetes. Endpoints included major clinical events that affect the life and well-being of patients, such as stroke, angina, heart attack, blindness, renal failure and amputations.

The trial was started in 1977 and recruited over 5000 patients. All were treated initially by diet and those who remained hyperglycaemic were randomly allocated to diet, sulphonylurea or insulin. Obese patients were also randomized to metformin. Patients who failed monotherapy with sulphonylurea were further randomized to combination therapy; those who failed monotherapy with metformin also received sulphonylurea, while those who developed hyperglycaemic symptoms or fasting hyperglycaemia on maximal oral therapy were transferred to insulin.[69] Results indicate that lowering raised blood glucose and blood pressure levels, with intensive use of existing treatments, substantially reduces the risk of heart disease, stroke and death from diabetes-related diseases as well as diabetic eye disease and early kidney damage. However, it is important to note that intensive treatment is not without side-effects. In the UKPDS, patients in the intensive group had more hypoglycaemic episodes compared with those in the conventional treatment group. In addition, weight gain was significantly higher in the intensive group and patients assigned insulin had a greater gain in weight compared with those on hypoglycaemic medication.

4.8   Quality of Life

Quality of life (QoL) is increasingly recognized as an important health outcome in its own right, and has been said to represent the ultimate goal of all health interventions.[70] More than 50 years ago, the World Health Organisation stated that health was defined not only by the absence of disease and infirmity, but also by the presence of physical, mental and social well-being.[71] Most studies report worse quality of life for people with diabetes compared with the general population, especially regarding physical functioning and well-being.[72,73] Snoek[74] suggests that one of the most intriguing findings from QoL research is the relatively weak association between patients' objective health status and their subjective life quality. Apparently, health in itself does not guarantee happiness, nor does good glycemic control. Studies examining the relationship between diabetes control (HbA1c) and subjective well-being find low correlations if any,[75–77] although there is evidence to suggest that patients suffering from diabetes-related complications on average report lower levels of QoL compared with patients without secondary complications.[78] Specific measures, such as the Problem Areas in Diabetes (PAID) scale and the Diabetes Quality of Life (DQOL) scale, can help health care professionals to identify areas of patient concern and worry and thereby serve as aids to assessment.

4.9   Management of Diabetes in Older Adults

The management of diabetes in the older adult poses a unique challenge. Several factors, including limited financial resources and coexisting diseases, complicate diabetes management. Accordingly, diabetes in older adults is often difficult to manage, and is often poorly or insufficiently treated.[79] The treatment targets for patients with type 2 diabetes should be the same as for type 1, namely to abolish diabetic symptoms and the risk of acute metabolic complications, to reduce the threat of chronic diabetic complications, to increase life expectancy to that of non-diabetic populations and to restore quality of life to normal. At present, none of these aims is met in a substantial proportion of cases.

The specifics of how to manage elderly patients with diabetes, prioritize their problems, and implement effective interventions for functional outcomes are not clear. For example, glycaemic control, management of blood pressure and hyperlipidaemia each could conceivably affect cognitive decline, but little research exists to inform clinicians. The association between diabetes and physical disabilities seems to be mediated by several potentially modifiable factors, including coronary heart disease, stroke, obesity, physical inactivity and depression. This would imply that prevention of secondary cardiovascular disease, weight loss, exercise programmes and screening for depression and its treatment may help prevent disability, but again there is a paucity of research relating such interventions to functional outcomes. It is also important to note that guidelines for the quality of care in diabetes are based primarily on research conducted among middle-aged populations, and their appropriateness in the face of complex complications related to ageing is less clear.

Treatment goals

A key step in developing a diabetes management programme for older adults with diabetes is to establish treatment goals. Management goals should be individualized. Each case should be subjected to a vigorous risk/benefit analysis. Several considerations should be taken into account, including the individual's functional capabilities and level of dependency when individual goals are set. Indeed, for individuals with high levels of dependency, the risks of hypoglycaemia may outweigh the benefits of tight glycaemic control. Unrealistic expectations for an older individual who has poor vision, poor dexterity, and no social support system are also counterproductive. All of these factors should be kept in mind. However, age per se should not be an excuse for denying optimal glycaemic control to older adults with diabetes.

Obesity and diabetes

Obesity is one of the biggest obstacles to the management of diabetes and makes a significant contribution to the morbidity and mortality associated with type 2 diabetes, largely through its contribution to cardiovascular disease. In non-diabetic individuals, obesity is commonly associated with hypertension, dyslipidaemia and ultimately atherogenesis and premature death from cardiovascular disease. These risks appear to be accentuated in people with diabetes. For example, the risk of premature death is 10-fold greater in a diabetic person with a BMI > 36, compared with a non-obese diabetic patient.

Managing a patient with type 2 diabetes and obesity can be seen as a conflict of interests, because the most effective treatments for type 2 diabetes, that is insulin and sulphonylureas, frequently lead to weight gain. This is one of the problems of the conventional approach to the management of diabetes in which the disease and its associated complications are considered separately. The side effects and metabolic effects of drugs used to manage diabetes frequently exacerbate the other complications. For example, if the physician focuses on achieving control of blood glucose levels with insulin or sulphonylurea therapy, this can lead to weight gain, which in turn may worsen insulin resistance and other aspects of the metabolic syndrome. Exacerbation of hypertension and dyslipidaemia may then arise.

In contrast to these approaches, recent studies have shown that addressing the problem of obesity first can lead to an improvement in blood glucose control, which can be accompanied by a decrease in blood pressure, an increase in insulin sensitivity and favourable changes in blood lipid profiles. Swedish and American studies of patients undergoing bariatric gastric surgery, for example, found that of the 50 per cent of patients who had type 2 diabetes or were glucose intolerant before surgery most developed normal glucose tolerance within 5–6 years of surgery.[80] Thus, the successful loss of a substantial amount of weight improved glucose tolerance dramatically.

Other studies have shown that a loss of 5–10 per cent of body weight can produce statistically significant benefits. Several studies have reported that patients achieving a loss of body weight of five per cent or greater achieved a small but significant decrease in HbA1c levels, and that clinically meaningful improvements in HbA1c can be obtained with a greater than 10 per cent decrease in body weight.[81,82] This is comparable, for example, to the improvement in glycaemic control anticipated following the addition of a second oral antidiabetic agent.

Weight loss in obese patients with diabetes can therefore significantly improve their clinical condition. As already emphasized, the multiple beneficial effects of weight loss on several features of the metabolic syndrome that contribute to atheroma mean that weight reduction is a rational and conceptually attractive option in the management of type 2 diabetes. Indeed, in theory at least, it could be preferable to using several different drugs to treat the individual disorders of this syndrome.

Lifestyle change

Lifestyle changes, especially dietary modification and increased physical activity are the starting point for many individuals. Recommendations are that high fat, high energy diets rich in refined carbohydrate should be replaced by a diet based on complex carbohydrates (accounting for over 50 per cent of total energy intake), with a low fat content (less than 30 per cent of total energy), especially saturated animal fats. The overweight majority with type 2 diabetes are also encouraged to lose weight to bring their body-mass index (BMI) down to an acceptable level ($<25\,kg/m^2$). Unfortunately, lifestyle measures achieve adequate blood glucose control (fasting blood glucose levels $<7\,mmol/l$) in only 10–20 per cent of cases.[83]

Diet

Dietary intervention has long been a cornerstone of diabetes management. Fundamental to any dietary recommendation is ensuring that essential dietary needs are met with adequate provision of vitamins and minerals. Two aspects of diet need to be addressed in any dietary programme: the total caloric intake, which is a key to maintenance of body weight or weight reduction; and dietary composition, or the distribution of fat, carbohydrate and protein calories.

There are a number of special issues to consider in dietary management of older adults with diabetes. Older adults with a significant mobility limitation may be relatively inactive and have low caloric utilization. Thus, caloric intake may need to be limited to rather low levels to achieve significant weight reduction. The potential benefit of caloric restriction and weight reduction under such circum- stances needs to be balanced against the potential risk for complications related to undernutrition. Such patients also may have difficulty with access to food both in terms of food preparation and shopping to bring food in. Furthermore, dietary habits established for a lifetime and often with a cultural background may be particularly difficult to modify. Older persons, especially men living alone, may have limited food preparation skills. The presence of impaired cognitive function may make following a dietary prescription particularly difficult. Any of these issues can be modified if there is sufficient caregiver support and/or social services that can assist with providing meals in the home setting.

Problems with taste and oral health, which are common in older people, may further limit adaptation to a prescribed dietary regimen. Oral health problems can be exacerbated by diabetes, which may increase the rate of periodontal disease. This may be a growing issue as more older adults are keeping their teeth for longer periods.

Physical activity

A programme of increased physical activity is an important adjunct to diabetes management. By increasing caloric expenditure, an exercise programme can facilitate the effectiveness of a weight reduction programme for overweight people with diabetes. It may also help prevent reaccumulation of weight following caloric-restriction-facilitated weight loss. Simple increases of physical activity, such as with stretching exercises or walking, are potentially useful to improve overall functional capability. There is also a growing body of evidence that exercise training can enhance sensitivity to insulin by improving insulin-mediated glucose uptake. Thus, exercise training may have a beneficial effect beyond simply enhancing the effectiveness of a weight reduction programme. Furthermore, patients with diabetes may benefit from the effects of exercise training to enhance cardiovascular function, lower blood pressure, improve the lipid profile and, importantly, enhance psychological well-being. Accordingly, exercise may be a useful adjunct to drug therapy and may well contribute to enhanced effectiveness of glucose-lowering agents. Given the high prevalence of coronary artery disease in older adults with diabetes, which may be asymptomatic or atypical in symptoms, it is important for such individuals to have medically supervised stress testing before entering any challenging exercise training programme. An additional issue to consider in an older person is the potential for foot and joint injury with upright exercise such as jogging. Particular attention should be given to the foot examination in an older person prior to and during the course of exercise training. Finally, because of its effects to enhance glucose uptake by muscle, exercise training may contribute to risk for hypoglycaemia in patients treated with hypoglycaemic agents.

The challenge of type 2 diabetes

The error in regarding type 2 as 'mild diabetes'[7] is now well recognized, as is its importance as a major cause of disability and premature death. These problems are accentuated by the very large numbers of individuals concerned, considerably more than those with type 1. In 1997, approximately 14 million Americans had diabetes, with over 700 000 new cases reported yearly.[84] Around 1.4 million people in the UK today have diabetes. At least a million more, 'the missing million', are thought to have diabetes that has not yet been diagnosed.[85] This increasing prevalence is probably linked to the current obesity epidemic and the high levels of sedentary lifestyles in westernized societies and it is predicted to continue to increase sharply as the population ages.[86] Because type 2 diabetes is associated with such problematic comorbid conditions in older adults, including a substantially increased risk for cardiovascular disease, reducing risk factors such as obesity and physical inactivity through lifestyle modification, or at the very least limiting the disability associated with them, is crucial to the long term health of individuals with type 2 diabetes.[87] Although difficult to implement, lifestyle modification programmes also raise the possibility that such measures may ultimately be able to contain the current epidemic of type 2 diabetes and limit the vast individual, social and financial damage that it will otherwise cause.

Diabetes education for older adults

Diabetes education is an integral aspect of all diabetes management, regardless of the individual's age. Diabetes education should be recognized as a lifelong commitment, for both patients, families and the interdisciplinary diabetes team.

Effective education starts with an assessment of educational needs and readiness to learn. Just as diabetes treatment needs to be individualized, so do educational needs. Many older people with diabetes have had no formal diabetes education, often despite years of living with diabetes. There may be many misconceptions, fears and/or myths that need to be explored or acknowledged. Health beliefs, culture and religious beliefs may also influence adherence to diabetes treatment and management plans.

It is important to utilize principles of adult learning when providing education to older adults with diabetes. These principles include recognizing previous experiences, using a variety of teaching methods, adapting teaching materials to accommodate learning (i.e. large print, additional time for practicing skills), using a variety of teaching materials, making the education relevant and actively including the person in the learning process.

Breaking more complicated skills/information into smaller, simpler steps may assist with retention and mastery. Providing opportunities to practice skills and ask questions, as well as providing positive feedback, are all important.

Further, since social isolation is a potent but little understood risk factor for morbidity and mortality, and its negative consequences are most profound among the elderly, one-to-one and group classes can provide needed socialization and support for older adults. Other factors that may influence learning include the ageing process, other medical conditions/medications and emotions. Including the family/caregivers in the assessment and education process is essential since they may be providing the care as well as reinforcing education/monitoring practices. Utilization of community resources (i.e. Meals on Wheels, local diabetes organizations for education and support groups, home care nurses/aides) is also important. Follow-up is essential to clarify questions and concerns as well as to encourage and motivate patients. Telephone follow-up may be more realistic in this regard due to problems of transportation and mobility in general.

Medication

Older adults with diabetes pose a particular challenge to clinicians with respect to managing medications. Not only are comorbidities common in this population group but also careful management of these comorbidities is perhaps more important than in patients without diabetes. While non-pharmacological interventions for managing diabetes and the associated comorbidities are integral to the treatment plan, in reality the cornerstone of management remains pharmacotherapy. As a consequence, there are strong factors that favour polypharmacy in older adults with diabetes.

Rational medication prescribing dictates that the fewest medications be used to achieve the therapeutic goals as determined by clinician and patient, and once-daily dosing is generally preferred. Multiple medications not only add to the cost and complexity of therapeutic regimens, but also place patients at greater risk for adverse drug reactions and drug–drug interactions. Studies evaluating appropriate prescribing in the elderly consistently find frequent polypharmacy and use of excessive or potentially harmful drugs. To address the problem of inappropriate polypharmacy, efforts have been studied in both inpatient and outpatient settings[88,89] to decrease use of unnecessary medications, as well as the overall number of medications, in both inpatient and outpatient settings.

Thus health care professionals caring for older people with diabetes face a therapeutic dilemma: balancing the needs of their patients and attempting to achieve optimum control of medical problems while trying to keep the medication profile as simple and small as possible.

Fear of hypoglycaemia

Many older adults with diabetes have considerable fear and anxiety about the possibility of hypoglycaemia and its negative consequences, and hypoglycaemic episodes are sometimes a major problem for many insulin-taking older adults. As well as placing patients at physical risk, hypoglycaemia can also result in serious psychological problems. These include extreme fear of hypoglycaemia and conflicts in relationships. Sometimes this fear can result in inappropriate self-treatment, such as behaviours that keep blood glucose levels in a higher, 'safer' range. In addition, family members, carers or spouses can also develop a fear of hypoglycaemia, and often show high levels of fear particularly if the older adult has experienced unconsciousness due to hypoglycaemia or had an episode when the spouse/carer was not present. This fear can create tension and conflict in relationships and carers and others close to the individual can become overprotective and hypervigilant, which may well be resented by the individual with diabetes.

Individuals with diabetes rely on symptoms to warn them that their blood glucose is too low. Because both the type and intensity of hypoglycaemic symptoms vary from one individual to another and across the lifespan, it is important to help older adults with diabetes to identify their own best warning cues. Health care professionals can objectively assess patients' symptoms by using a blood glucose monitoring diary in which patients/carers record symptoms along with their blood glucose test results. Arming patients with knowledge and providing them with the learning experience of blood glucose monitoring diaries can be a significant aid in patients' awareness and understanding about how their bodies respond to hypoglycaemia. With this, patients who are vulnerable can potentially learn to reduce both the fear and the occurrence of hypoglycaemic episodes.

4.10   Self-Management Issues

Diabetes treatment predominantly involves self-management behaviours on the part of the patient, which include daily injections and medication taking, glucose testing and the modification of physical activity and dietary habits. Problems in following diabetes regimens have been well documented[90,91] and these problems can be further exacerbated in older and more frail individuals. Research has consistently found that while the various diabetes self-care behaviours are relatively independent of one another[92] dietary aspects of the regime are experienced as the most difficult followed by physical activity.[93–95] Most patients find medication taking to be the area in which they have the least difficulty,[96] which may be because this is the regimen area emphasized most by health care professionals and most associated with 'managing an illness' in the public's perception.

Educational and psychosocial interventions

Since implementing diabetes management lies largely with the patient's daily efforts,[97,98] numerous patient education interventions have been developed. These interventions were systematically reviewed in two meta-analyses[99,100] and have been shown to improve self-care and health status, a finding that was recently reinforced by a survey of educational and psychosocial interventions for people with diabetes.[101] Several patient activation interventions have reported strong and wide ranging effects including improvements in self-efficacy, metabolic control, patient satisfaction and quality of life.[102–104] Controlled studies have demonstrated lasting improvements in quality of life as well as glycaemic control.[105,106] These benefits have also been accomplished with minority and older individuals.[107,102] In addition, tailored nutrition messages have been shown to be effective in promoting dietary fat reduction[108,109] and physical activity.[110] Computer-tailored interventions are also proving increasingly efficient and effective in motivating people to adopt health-promoting behaviours.[111,112]

Lifestyle modification interventions

Lifestyle modification interventions, which focus on changing behaviours which are thought to contribute to, or maintain, obesity and inactivity, have their roots in behavioural modification and include the use of self-monitoring and goal setting, stimulus control and modification of eating style and habits, the use of reinforcement of healthy behaviours, cognitive behavioural therapy interventions that focus on identifying barriers to change and improving coping skills, relapse prevention training and maintenance and the use of social support. All of these strategies focus on changing the diabetic individual's problematic dietary habits and physical inactivity in order to reduce obesity and increase physical activity, both of which have been shown to improve health outcomes in individuals with diabetes.

Social support

Social support is an important component of successful lifestyle change. Many studies have found that individuals with higher levels of social support tend to do better.[113–115] Social support may involve including the family in the intervention, participation in a community-based programme or involvement in any outside social activity. Peer and family support may be particularly useful because it helps patients learn greater self-acceptance, develop new norms for interpersonal relationships and manage stressful situations.[116]

   Not everyone receives the social support they need. Many factors determine whether people receive support and people's need for, sources of and ability to provide social support change throughout the life span.[117] Importantly, old age is a time when social support sometimes declines. A steadily increasing number of older people are living alone and are therefore more likely to experience social isolation and this has important implications for older adults with diabetes. Although people's social networks do not get smaller in old age, the elderly exchange less support, perhaps because of the loss of a spouse, or because they may feel reluctant to ask for help if they become unable to reciprocate.

4.11   Practice Implications

Assessment

Diabetes mellitus in older adults is a complex disorder that can have effects on many body systems, and its treatment may require a complex programme including medication plus lifestyle changes. The choice of intervention strategies and the patient's capability to adhere to a diabetes treatment programme may be limited by the presence of other health problems, as well as by the patient's living situation, economic status and indeed availability of caregiver support. A comprehensive assessment is therefore highly appropriate to provide the basis for developing a treatment plan for an older person with diabetes.

Medical assessment

Once a diagnosis of diabetes is established, a thorough medical evaluation is needed. Since the risk of developing diabetes complications is related to the duration of hyperglycaemia, efforts should be made to pinpoint the time of onset. However, because of the usual uncertainty about time of onset, a careful search for existing diabetes complications is warranted even when a new diagnosis is made in an older adult. Such an evaluation is equally justified in a patient with a history of diabetes who is establishing a new relationship with a health care system or primary care provider.

The medical evaluation of an older adult with diabetes should also include information about other coexisting risk factors including hypertension, hyperlipidaemia and smoking. These conditions interact with diabetes to increase risk of adverse cardiovascular events and therefore need to be addressed in an overall patient management programme. The drug history of an older adult with diabetes is important both to identify drug therapy that may be contributing to the patient's hyperglycaemia and to identify potential drug interactions that may affect diabetes management. The initial assessment should also include a diet history, a review of potential nutritional problems and an oral health assessment, as dietary intervention is a key component of a treatment programme for virtually all patients with diabetes. Particular attention should be paid to dietary habits, ethnic food preferences and meal patterns.

Assessment of personal models of diabetes

Personal models of illness are people's beliefs and emotions about their disease. In the same way that people have beliefs about health, they also have beliefs about illness. Psychologists have shown that these beliefs appear to follow a pattern and are made up of (1) identity, for example the diagnosis and symptoms, (2) consequences, for example, beliefs about seriousness, (3) time line, for example, how long will it last, (4) cause, for example, due to eating too much sugar, a virus, and (5) cure/control, for example, whether the condition requires medical intervention.

Of the many beliefs that patients hold about their illness, two may relate to long term adjustment: beliefs about the cause of their illness ('Why did it happen?') and beliefs about whether or not the illness can be controlled ('What can I do to manage it now?').

Why did it happen?

A large number of researchers have noted that people suffering from both acute and chronic illness develop theories about where their illnesses came from. Individuals' theories about the origins of chronic illnesses, such as diabetes, include stress, physical injury, disease-causing bacteria and God's will. Importantly, where people place the blame for their illness is highly significant. Do they blame themselves, another person, the environment or a quirk of fate?

Self-blame for chronic illness is widespread. People frequently perceive themselves as having brought on their diabetes by their own actions. In some cases, these perceptions are to some extent correct. Poor health habits such as smoking, improper diet or lack of exercise can cause illnesses like heart disease, for example. But what are the consequences of self-blame? Unfortunately, there is no straightforward answer to this question. Some researchers suggest that self-blame can lead to guilt, self-recrimination or depression. Self-blaming individuals may be poorly adjusted to their illness because they focus on things they could have or should have done to prevent it. On the other hand, other research suggests that self-blame may be adaptive. Perceiving the cause as self-generated may represent an effort to assume control over the disorder; such feelings can be adaptive in coping with and coming to terms with the disorder. It may be that self-blame may be adaptive under certain conditions and not under others.

Understanding the implications

Understanding the cause of the illness and developing an insight into the implications of the illness gives the illness meaning. A sense of meaning contributes to the process of coping and adapting to diabetes.

What can I do to manage it now?

Researchers have also examined whether patients who believe they can control their diabetes are better off than those who do not see their diabetes as under their control, and people develop a number of control-related beliefs with respect to their condition. A sense of control can be achieved either through psychological techniques such as developing a positive attitude, meditation, self-hypnosis or a type of causal attribution, or through behavioural techniques such as changing diet, changing medications, accessing information or controlling any side effects. These processes contribute to a sense of 'mastery' over the diabetes.

Assessment of diabetes knowledge

Because of the complexity of diabetes management, usually requiring both lifestyle and medication interventions, the patient and caregivers must be actively involved in their own care and take as much responsibility for its many aspects as possible. It is particularly important to review the individual's knowledge base regarding diabetes and its complications. The diabetes education programme that becomes part of the treatment plan can then provide this knowledge base for new patients or fill in needed gaps for existing patients.

Assessment of functional status

A review of activities of daily living and instrumental activities of daily living should also be a part of comprehensive assessment of an older adult with diabetes. Diabetes puts the individual at increased risk for functional deficits. Such functional limitations must also be considered in developing a diabetes treatment program. In addition to general assessment of functional status, the ability of the patient and caregiver to carry out diabetes-specific functional tasks needs to be evaluated. For example, the ability to carry out home glucose monitoring or self-injection of insulin requires certain functional abilities.

Assessment of psychological status

Cognitive status

There are numerous published neuropsychological tests, which can help assess an individual's cognitive status, ranging from premorbid intelligence to visuo-spatial coordination to abstract reasoning. The difficulty in choosing what test to use and how to assess cognitive function in diabetes arises from the fact that none of these tests has been specifically developed with the diabetes patient in mind and that there is much uncertainty as to what cognitive skills diabetes is likely to adversely affect. Assuming however that the purpose of the assessment was to gauge whether self-care is likely to be compromised as a result of possible cognitive decline in older patients with type 2 diabetes, it is proposed that tests assessing specific cognitive processes relevant to self-care (rather than overall functioning) may well be useful. Tasks such as implicit and explicit memory as well as problem solving are likely to be useful in negotiating and following through self-care plans and as such should perhaps be routinely assessed.

Depression and anxiety

These conditions are easily screened for by using standard, quick and easy to administer and score questionnaires. The Hospital Anxiety and Depression Scale[118] and the Zung Self Rating Anxiety Questionnaire (ZSRA)[119] as well as Beck's Depression Inventory (BDI)[120] and the CES-D[121] have all successfully been used with patients with diabetes in the past. All are self-report measures, are scored by use of a simple scoring key and, alongside a diagnostic interview, can be used to identify patients with elevated symptoms of depression, anxiety or both.

Psychosocial assessment

Research suggests that adherence to medical recommendations tends to be low when the regimen is complex, must be followed for a long time, requires changes in the person's lifestyle and is designed to prevent rather than cure illness. Treatment regimens for diabetes have all of these characteristics. In addition, psychosocial factors in older patients' lives are related to adherence to treatment.

Two of these factors are social support and self-efficacy. A study of type 2 individuals found that self-reports of adherence to the dietary, exercise and glucose testing aspects of their regimens increased with their perceived social support.[122] However, the role of social support is unclear because it was not related to actual glucose control, as measured by analysis of blood samples. Other research has shown that diabetes self-efficacy for being able to follow the diabetes regimen is related to self-reports of subsequent adherence and their actual glucose control.[123,124]

Coping processes are also important in diabetes care. Stress impairs blood sugar control in many individuals with diabetes,[125] especially those who have sedentary lifestyles.[126] The effects of stress may occur in two ways. First, when people are under stress, the adrenal glands release epinephrine and cortisol into the bloodstream.[127] Epinephrine causes the pancreas to decrease insulin production; cortisol causes the liver to increase glucose production and body tissues to decrease their use of glucose. These biochemical reactions to stress clearly worsen the glucose regulation problems of individuals with diabetes. Second, stress can affect blood glucose levels indirectly by reducing adherence to diabetes regimens.[128] Many older adults with diabetes do not cope well with their condition and suffer from severe depression.[129,130] The more the condition interferes with their daily activities and reduces their feelings of personal control, the more depressed they feel.[131]

People's everyday lives present many circumstances that make it difficult to adhere to diabetes regimens.[132] Individuals with diabetes may feel that testing their glucose levels at work or school is embarrassing, or forget to take their testing materials with them, or have difficulty getting up on weekend mornings to take their injections on time, or make mistakes in judgments about what they can eat, for example.

A number of other issues can be important. First, because some temporary weight gain tends to occur when people with diabetes get their glucose under control, many female patients, in an effort to control their weight, fail to take their insulin.[133] Second, a regimen's dietary recommendations may be incompatible with the food habits of patients in certain ethnic groups.[134] Third, individuals with diabetes often feel frustrated when they 'didn't cheat', but their glucose control is off target for some other reason, such as being under stress. Fourth, because diabetes is not a painful condition, patients may feel that following the regimen closely is not critical.[135]

One other psychosocial situation that can lead to diminished adherence is when the patient and the health care professional have different goals of treatment. That such differences exist has been demonstrated in a number of studies. Parkin and Skinner,[136] for example, have demonstrated in a study concerned with communication processes in the consultation that patients and professionals in a specialist centre completely disagreed on issues discussed in the consultation 20 per cent of the time, patients and professionals disagreed on the decisions made in the consultation 21 per cent of the time and, importantly, patients and professionals disagreed on the goals set 45 per cent of the time.

Similarly, results from a study to investigate differences in diabetes beliefs and attitudes between patients and health care professionals involved in their care[137] suggest significant discrepancies in diabetes perspectives. The finding that the attitudes of all of the health care professionals towards the seriousness of type 2 diabetes differed significantly from those of the patients in this study is of particular interest, and this discrepancy between health care professional and patient perceptions is reflected in previous research. Larme and Pugh[138] for example suggest that provider urgency to control diabetes contrasts sharply with patient experience and awareness. It is suggested that the lack of dramatic symptoms to 'scare' patients and the lack of public health campaigns to bring the seriousness of diabetes to patients' attention (such as for hypertension, cholesterol and smoking), combined with cultural and economic barriers, mean that patients neither take diabetes seriously nor listen to their health care professionals. It is also possible that patients' views may reflect the manner in which health care professionals who wish to maintain a therapeutic relationship with patients that is reassuring and encouraging convey information about the seriousness of type 2 diabetes. A number of other possible explanations for this discrepancy in perceptions of the seriousness of diabetes have also been suggested. For example, the health care professionals' sense of urgency to control diabetes is heightened by their knowledge that the consequences are devastating if patients do not follow their recommendations, especially about lifestyle changes, and they are aware that they are treating an underlying condition affecting the entire body, and not just treating symptoms.

While the patients in this study agreed that type 2 diabetes was a serious disease, the strength of their agreement was relatively weak. This finding has important implications for patient education and intervention. The literature on adherence to diabetes treatment regimens for example suggests that beliefs about the serious-ness of type 2 diabetes are strongly related to adherence to treatment,[139] metabolic control[140] and self-management behaviours.[141] Diabetes requires difficult and long-lasting behaviour changes on the part of patients and it is unlikely that such changes will be made and sustained unless patients and health care professionals are in agreement about the serious nature of this illness.

These findings then have significant implications for forming collaborative alliances with patients and highlight the need to recognize the distinctions and discrepancies between practitioner and patient perspectives in diabetes which may potentially impact health outcomes.

4.12 Summary and Conclusions

Transitions across the lifespan are reflected in changing patterns of health and illness behaviours. These patterns are moderated by biological ageing, by pathologies and life experiences and also by the changing personal affective coping strategies, the psychosocial context, the family and the social network. These complex inter-relationships have implications for illness representations and for selection of coping responses to treatment regimens in diabetes. In addition, there are different expectations and response patterns anticipated from different disease entities across the adult lifespan. Health psychology has contributed to our understanding of these changes in three major areas. First, it is clear that a variety of specific tactics or procedures for symptom evaluation may encourage benign attributions and delay in seeking care. These include attributing slow-to-develop symptoms to ageing, ambiguous symptoms to stress and the minimization of perceived severity of shared symptoms, an effect more likely among the older persons who are also multi-symptomatic. In diabetes, these changes are potentially risk inducing as many of the life-threatening complications which are most prevalent during the later years are slow to develop and ambiguous in presentation.

As the number of older people with diabetes and other chronic diseases increases, outcomes such as cognitive and physical disability will become greater concerns because of their implications for quality of life, loss of independence and demands on caregivers. The management of these patients will be complex because they may have several other diseases and require numerous medications, compounded by the fact that at least half of older diabetic adults will have a major physical or cognitive disability. Health care practitioners will need to be aware of the implications of diabetes in older adults as they assess and prioritize treatment for the individual patient. This will require public health agencies and diabetes research programmes to adapt to the shifting demographics of the disease, by more directly examining the effects of diabetes and interventions on the outcomes that are most important to older adults with diabetes.

References

1. Gatling W, Houston AC, Hill RD. An epidemiological survey: the prevalence of diabetes mellitus in a typical English community. *J R College Physicians London* 1985; **4**: 248–250.
2. Zimmet P. Type 2 (non-insulin-dependent diabetes) – an epidemiological overview. *Diabetologia* 1982; **22**: 399–411.
3. Zimmet P. Challenges in diabetes epidemiology – from West to the rest. *Diabetes Care* 1992; **15**: 232–252.
4. Mather HM, Keen H. The Southall Diabetes Survey; prevalence of known diabetes in Asians and Europeans. *BMJ* 1985; **291**: 1081–1084.
5. Rendell M. C-peptide levels as a criterion in the treatment of maturity-onset diabetes. *J Clin Endocrinol Metab* 1983; **57**: 1198–1206.
6. Cohen M, Crosbie C, Cusworth L, Aimmet P. Insulin – not always a life sentence; withdrawal of insulin therapy in non-insulin-dependent diabetes. *Diabetes Res* 1984; **1**: 31–34.
7. Gill GC. Type 2 diabetes – is it 'mild diabetes'? *Practical Diabetes* 1986; **3**: 280–282.
8. Mayfield JA, Deb P, Potter DEB. Diabetes and long-term care. In *Diabetes in America*, 2nd edn, Publication No. 95-1468. Bethesda, MD: NIH, 1995, pp 571–586.

9. Sinclair AJ, Gadsby R, Penfold S, Croxson SCM, Bayer AJ. Prevalence of diabetes in care home residents. *Diabetes Care* 2001; **24**(6): 1066–1068.

10. Benbow SJ, Walsh A, Gill GV. Diabetes in the institutionalised elderly: a forgotten population? *BMJ* 1997; **315**: 1868–1870.

11. *National Population Projections: 2000-based*. National Statistics, © Crown Copyright 2002 (actual and projected population by age, UK, 2000–2025).

12. Kane RL, Ouslander JG, Abrass IB. *Essentials of Clinical Geriatrics*, 3rd edn. New York: McGraw-Hill, 1994.

13. Miller RA. The biology of aging and longevity. In Hazzard WL, Bierman EL, Blass JP, Ettinger WH, Halter JB, Andres R. (eds), *Principles of Geriatric Medicine and Gerontology*, 3rd edn. New York: McGraw-Hill, 1994 Chapter 1, pp 3–15.

14. Salthouse TA. *Theoretical Perspectives on Cognitive Aging*. Hillsdale, NJ: Erlbaum, 1991.

15. Lezak MD. *Neuropsychological Assessment*. Oxford: Oxford University Press, 1995.

16. Kart C. Experiencing symptoms: attribution and misattribution of illness among the aged. In Haug MR. (ed.), *Elderly Patients and Their Doctors*. New York: Springer, 1981, pp 70–78.

17. Brody EM, Kleban MH. Physical and mental health symptoms of older people: who do they tell? *J Am Geriatr Soc* 1981; **29**: 442–449.

18. Leventhal H, Diefenbach M. The active side of illness cognition. In Skelton JA, Croyle RT. (eds), *Mental Representation in Health and Illness*. New York: Springer, 1991, pp 247–272.

19. Prohaska TR, Keller ML, Leventhal EA, Leventhal H. Impact of symptoms and aging attribution on emotions and coping. *Health Psychol* 1987; **6**: 495–514.

20. Keller ML, Leventhal H, Prohaska TR, Leventhal EA. Beliefs about aging and illness in a community sample. *Res Nursing Health* 1989; **12**: 247–255.

21. Tun P, Perlmuter LC, Russo PA, Nathan DM. Memory self-assessment and performance in aged diabetics and non-diabetics. *Exp Aging Res* 1987; **13** (3): 151–157.

22. Asimakopoulou KG, Hampson SE. Cognitive function and diabetes self management in older patients with type 2 diabetes. *Diabetes Spectrum* 2002; **15**: 116–121.

23. Fujimoto WY. A national multicenter study to learn whether type II diabetes can be prevented: The Diabetes Prevention Program. *Clin Diabetes* 1997; January/February: 13–15.

24. Barrett-Connor E, Criqui MH, Klauber MR, Holdbook M. Diabetes and hypertension in a community of older adults. *Am J Epidemiol* 1981; **113**: 276–284.

25. Reaven GM. Role of insulin resistance in human disease. *Diabetes* 1988; **37**: 1595–1607.

26. UKPDS Group. United Kingdom Prospective Diabetes Study. Intensive blood-glucose control with sulphonylureas or insulin compared with conventional treatment and risk of complications in patients with type 2 diabetes (UKPDS 33). *Lancet* 1998; **352**: 837–853.

27. Bjorntorp P. Abdominal obesity and the development of non-insulin-dependent diabetes mellitus. *Diabetes Metab Rev* 1988; **4**: 615–622.

28. Marks HH, Krall LP. Onset, course, prognosis and mortality of diabetes mellitus. In Marble A, Proctor E (eds), *Joslin's Diabetes Mellitus*, 11th edn. Philadelphia PA: Lea and Febiger, 1971, pp 209–254.

29. Rytter L, Troelsen S, Beck-Nielsen H. Prevalence and mortality of acute myocardial infarction in patients with diabetes. *Diabetes Care* 1985; **8**: 230–234.

30. Gwilt D. Why do diabetic patients die after myocardial infarction? *Practical Diabetes* 1984; **1**: 36–39.

31. Watkins PJ, Grenfell A, Edmonds M. Diabetic complications of non-insulin dependent diabetes. *Diabet Med* 1987; **4**: 293–296.

32. McCulloch DK, Campbell IW, Wu FC, Prescott RJ, Clarke BF. The prevalence of diabetic impotence. *Diabetologia* 1980; **18**: 279–283.

33. Strachan MW, Deary IJ, Ewing FME, Frier BM. Is Type II diabetes associated with increased risk of cognitive dysfunction? *Diabetes Care* 1997; **20** (3): 438–445.
34. Asimakopoulou KG, Hampson SE, Morrish NJ. Neuropsychological functioning in older people with type 2 diabetes: the effect of controlling for confounding factors. *Diabet Med* 2002; **19**(4): 311–316.
35. Perlmuter LC, Hakami MK, Hodgson Harrington C, Ginsberg J, *et al.* Decreased cognitive function in aging non-insulin-dependent diabetic patients. *Am J Med* 1984; **77**(6): 1043–1048.
36. Reaven GM, Thompson L, Nahum D, Haskins E. Relationship between hyperglycemia and cognitive function in older NIDDM patients. *Diabetes Care* 1990; **13** (1): 16–21.
37. Biessels GJ, ter Braak EWMT, Erkelens DW, Hijman R. Cognitive function in patients with type 2 diabetes mellitus, *Neurosci Res Commun* 2001; **28** (1): 11–22.
38. Ryan CM, Geckle M. Why is learning and memory dysfunction in type 2 diabetes limited to older adults? *Diabetes Metab Res Rev* 2000; **16**: 308–315.
39. Jagusch W, Cramon DYV, Renner R, Hepp KD. Cognitive function and metabolic state in elderly diabetic patients. *Diabetes Nutr Metab* 1992; **5**: 265–274.
40. Gregg EG, Yaffe K, Cauley JA, Rolka DB, Blackwell TL, Narayan KMV, Cummings SR. Is diabetes associated with cognitive impairment and cognitive decline among older women? *Arch Intern Med* 2000; **160**: 174–179.
41. Allen KV, Frier BM, Strachan MWJ. The relationship between type 2 diabetes and cognitive dysfunction: longitudinal studies and their methodological limitations. *Eur J Pharmacol* 2004; **490**: 169–175.
42. Fontbonne A, Berr C, Ducimetiere PD, Alperovitch A. Changes in cognitive abilities over a 4 year period are unfavourably affected in elderly diabetic subjects. *Diabetes Care* 2001; **24**: 2065–2070.
43. Haan MM, Shemanski L, Jagust WJ, Manolio TA, Kuller K. The role of APOE ε4 in modulating effects of other risk factors for cognitive decline in elderly persons. *JAMA* 1999; **282**: 40–46.
44. Sinclair AJ, Girling AJ, Bayer AJ. Cognitive dysfunction in older subjects with diabetes mellitus: impact on diabetes self-management and use of care services. *Diabetes Res Clin Practice* 2000; **50** (3): 203–212.
45. Goldberg JH, Breckenridge JN, Sheikh JI. Age differences in symptoms of depression and anxiety: examining behavioural medicine outpatients. *J Behavioral Med* 2003; **26** (2): 119–132.
46. Nickel JT, Brown KJ, Smith BA. Depression and anxiety among chronically ill heart patients: age differences in risk predictors. *Res Nursing Health* 1990; **13** (2): 87–97.
47. Kessing LV, Nilsson FM, Siersma V, Andersen PK. No increased risk of developing depression in diabetes compared to other chronic illness. *Diabetes Res Clin Practice* 2003; **62** (2): 113–121.
48. Nichols GA, Brown JB. Unadjusted and adjusted prevalence of diagnosed depression in type 2 diabetes. *Diabetes Care* 2003; **26** (3): 744–749.
49. De Groot M, Anderson R, Freedland KE, Clouse RE, Lustman PJ. Association of depression and diabetes complications: a meta-analysis. *Psychosomat Med* 2001; **63** (4): 619–630.
50. Pouwer F, Beekman AT, Nijpels G, Dekker JM, Snoek FJ, Kostense PJ, Heine RJ, Deeg DJ. Rates and risks for co-morbid depression in patients with type 2 diabetes mellitus: results from a community-based study. *Diabetologia* 2003; **46** (7): 892–898.
51. Snoek FJ, Skinner TC. Psychological counselling in problematic diabetes: does it help? *Diabet Med* 2002; **19**: 265–273.
52. McKellar JD, Humphreys K, Piette JD. Depression increases diabetes symptoms by complicating patients' self-care adherence. *Diabetes Educator* 2004; **30** (3): 485–492.

53. Piette JD, Richardson C, Valenstein M. Addressing the needs of patients with multiple chronic illnesses: the case of diabetes and depression. *American Journal of Managed Care* 2004; **110** (2, part 2): 152–162.

54. Kohen D, Burgess AP, Catalan J, Lant A. The role of anxiety and depression in quality of life and symptom reporting in people with diabetes mellitus. *Quality Life Res* 1998; **7** (3): 197–204.

55. Williams JW Jr, Katon W, Lin EH, Noel PH, Worchel J, Cornell J, Harpole L, Fultz BA, Hunkeler E, Mika VS, Unutzer J. The effectiveness of depression care management on diabetes-related outcomes in older patients. *Ann Intern Med* 2004; **140** (12): 1054–1056.

56. Lustman PJ, Griffin LS, Freedland KE, Kissel SS, Clouse RE. Cognitive behaviour therapy for depression in type 2 diabetes mellitus. A randomised controlled trial. *Ann Intern Med* 1998; **129** (8): 613–621.

57. Grigsby AB, Anderson RJ, Freedland KE, Clouse RE, Lustman PJ. Prevalence of anxiety in adults with diabetes. A systematic review. *J Psychosomat Res* 2002; **53**: 1053–1060.

58. Gregg EW, Beckles GL, Williamson DF, Leveille SG, Langlois JA, Engelgau MM. Diabetes and physical disability among US adults. *Diabetes Care* 2000; **23**: 1272–1277.

59. Gregg EW, Mangione CM, Cauley JA, Thompson TJ, Schwartz AV, Ensrud KE *et al.* Diabetes and incidence of functional disability in older women. *Diabetes Care* 2002; **25**: 61–67.

60. Schwartz AV, Sellmeyer DE, Ensrud KE, Cauley JA, Tabor HK, Schreiner PJ *et al.* Older women with diabetes have an increased risk of fracture: a prospective study. *J Clin Endocrinol Metab* 2001; **86**: 32–38.

61. Volpato S, Blaum C, Resnick H, Ferrucci L, Fried LP, Guralnik JM. Comorbidities and impairments explaining the association between diabetes and lower extremity disability. *Diabetes Care* 2002; **25**: 678–683.

62. Panzram G. Mortality and survival in Type 2 (non-insulin-dependent) diabetes mellitus. *Diabetologia* 1987; **30**: 123–131.

63. Goodkin G. Mortality factors in diabetes. *J Occupational Med* 1975; **17**: 716–721.

64. Nathan DM, Singer DE, Godine JE, Perlmutter LC. Non-insulin-dependent diabetes in older patients. Complications and risk factors. *Am J Med* 1986; **81**: 837–842.

65. Williams G. Management of non-insulin-dependent diabetes mellitus. *Lancet* 1994; **343**: 95–100.

66. Klein R, Klein BEK, Moss SE, David MD, DeMets DL. Glycosylated hemoglobin predicts the incidence and progression of diabetic retinopathy. *JAMA* 1988; **260**: 2864–2871.

67. Liu QZ, Knowler WC, Nelson RG *et al.* Insulin treatment, endogenous insulin concentration, and ECG abnormalities in diabetic Pima Indians. Cross-sectional and prospective analyses. *Diabetes* 1992; **41**: 1141–1150.

68. Klein R. Hyperglycaemia and microvascular and macrovascular disease in diabetes. *Diabetes Care* 1995; **18**: 258–271.

69. UKPDS Group. United Kingdom Prospective Diabetes Study. Intensive blood-glucose control with sulphonylureas or insulin compared with conventional treatment and risk of complications in patients with type 2 diabetes (UKPDS 33). *Lancet* 1998; **352**: 837–853.

70. Rubin RR. Diabetes and quality of life. *Diabetes Spectrum* 2000; **13**: 21–23.

71. World Health Organization. *Constitution of the World Health Organization.* Basic Documents. Geneva: World Health Organization, 1948.

72. Rubin RR, Peyrot M. Quality of life and diabetes. *Diabetes Metab Res Rev* 1999; **15**: 205–218.

73. Peyrot M, Rubin RR. Levels and risks of depression and anxiety symptomatology among diabetic adults. *Diabetes Care* 1997; **20**: 585–590.

74. Snoek FJ. Quality of life: a closer look at measuring patients' well-being. *Diabetes Spectrum* 2000; **13**: 24–28.

75. Nerenz DR, Repasky D, Whitehouse FW, Kahkonen DM. Ongoing assessment of health status in patients with diabetes mellitus. *Med Care* 1992; **5** (Suppl.): MS112–MS124.

76. Sonnaville JJ, Snoek FJ, Colly LP, Deville W, Wijkel D, Heine RJ. Well-being and symptoms in relation to insulin therapy in type 2 diabetes. *Diabetes Care* 1998; **6**: 919–924.

77. Weinberger M, Kirkman S, Samsa GP, Cowper PA, Shortliffe EA, Simel DL, Freussner JR. The relationship between glycemic control and health-related quality of life in patients with non-insulin dependent diabetes mellitus. *Medical Care* 1994; **12**: 1173–1181.

78. Klein BEK, Klein R, Moss SE. Self-rated health and diabetes of long duration: the Wisconsin Epidemiologic Study of Diabetic Retinopathy. *Diabetes Care* 1998; **21**: 236–240.

79. Williams G. Management of non-insulin-dependent diabetes mellitus. *Lancet* 1994; **343**: 95–100.

80. Pories WJ, Swanson MS, MacDonald KG. Who would have thought it – an operation proves to be the most effective therapy for adult-onset diabetes mellitus. *Ann Surg* 1995; **222**: 339–352.

81. UKPDS Group. United Kingdom Prospective Diabetes Study. Relative efficacy of randomly allocated diet, sulphonylurea, insulin, or metformin in patients with newly diagnosed noninsulin dependent diabetes followed for three years. *BMJ* 1995; **310**: 83–88.

82. Wing RR, Koeske R, Epstein LH, Norwalk MP, Gooding W, Becker D. Long term effects of modest weight loss in type 2 diabetic subjects. *Arch Intern Med* 1987; **147**: 1749–1753.

83. UKPDS Group. United Kingdom Prospective Diabetes Study. Intensive blood-glucose control with sulphonylureas or insulin compared with conventional treatment and risk of complications in patients with type 2 diabetes (UKPDS 33). *Lancet* 1998; **352**: 837–853.

84. Harris MI, Flegal KM, Cowie CC, Eberhardt MX, Goldstein DE, Little RR, Wiedmeyer H-M, Byrd-Holt DD. Prevalence of diabetes, impaired fasting glucose, and impaired glucose tolerance in U.S. adults: the Third National Health and Nutrition Examination Survey, 1988–1994. *Diabetes Care* 1998; **21**: 518–524.

85. British Diabetic Association. *Fact Sheet*. London: BDA, 2000.

86. Laws A, Reaven GM. Physical activity, glucose tolerance, and diabetes in older adults. *Ann Behav Med* 1991; **13**: 125–132.

87. Albu J, Pi-Sunyer FX. Obesity and diabetes. In Bray GA, Bouchard C, James WPT (eds), *Handbook of Obesity.*, New York: Dekker, 1998; pp 697–707.

88. Shad MU, Carmichael C, Preskorn SH, Horst DW. Prevalence of polypharmacy in different clinical settings and its relation to drug interactions. Presented at the 1999 Annual Meeting of the American Psychiatric Association, Washington, DC. 1999.

89. Reunanen A, Kangas T, Martikainen J, Klaukka T. Nationwide survey of comorbidity, use, and costs of all medications in Finnish diabetic individuals. *Diabetes Care* 2000; **23**: 1265–1271.

90. Glasgow RE. Compliance to diabetes regimens: conceptualization, complexity, and determinants. In Cramer JA, Spilker B (eds), *Patient Compliance in Medical Practice and Clinical Trials*. New York: Raven, 1991, pp 209–221.

91. Johnson SB. Health behavior and health status: concepts, methods and applications. *J Pediatr Psychol* 1994; **19**: 129–141.

92. Rubin RR, Peyrot M, Saudek CD. Effect of diabetes education on self-care, metabolic control, and emotional well-being. *Diabetes Care* 1989; **12**: 673–679.

93. Fisher EB Jr, Arfken CL, Heins JM, Houston CA, Jeffe DB, Sykes RK. Acceptance of diabetes in adults. In Gochman DS (ed.), *Handbook of Health Behavior Research II: Provider Determinants*. New York: Plenum, 1997, pp 189–212.

94. Ary DV, Toobert D, Wilson W, Glasgow R. Patient perspective on factors contributing to nonadherence to diabetes regimen. *Diabetes Care* 1986; **9**: 168–172.

95. Schlundt DG, Rea MR, Kline SS, Pichert JW. Situational obstacles to dietary adherence for adults with diabetes. *J Am Dietet Assoc* 1994; **94**: 874–876.

96. Glasgow RE. Social–environmental factors in diabetes: barriers to diabetes self-care. In Bradley C (ed.), *Handbook of Psychology and Diabetes*. Switzerland: Harwood, 1994, pp 335–349.

97. Eakin EG, Glasgow RE. The physician's role in diabetes self-management: helping patients to help themselves. *Endocrinologist* 1996; **6**: 1–10.

98. Anderson RM, Funnell MM, Barr PA, Dedrick RF, Davis WK. Learning to empower patients: results of a professional education program for diabetes educators. *Diabetes Care* 1991; **14**: 584–590.

99. Padgett D, Mumford E, Hynes M, Carter R. Meta-analysis of the effects of educational and psychosocial interventions on management of diabetes mellitus. *J Clin Epidemiol* 1988; **41**: 1007–1029.

100. Brown SA. Studies of educational interventions and outcomes in diabetic adults: a meta-analysis revisited. *Patient Education Counseling* 1990; **16**: 189–215.

101. Griffin S, Kinmouth AL, Skinner C, Kelly JC. *Educational and Psychosocial Interventions for Adults with Diabetes: a Survey of the Range and Types of Interventions, the Extent to Which they Have Been Evaluated in Controlled Trials and a Description of Their Relative Effectiveness as Reported in Existing Reviews*. London: British Diabetic Association, 1999.

102. Anderson RM, Herman WH, Davis JM, Friedman RP, Funnell MM. Neighbours HW. Barriers to improving diabetes care for black persons. *Diabetes Care* 1991; **14**: 605–609.

103. Anderson RM, Funnell MM, Butler PM, Arnold MS, Fitzgerald JT, Feste CC. Patient empowerment. Results of a randomized controlled trial. *Diabetes Care* 1995; **18**: 943–949.

104. Greenfield S, Kaplan SH, Ware JE, Yano EM, Frank H. Patients' participation in medical care: effects on blood sugar control and quality of life in diabetes. *J Gen Intern Med* 1988; **3**: 448–457.

105. Rubin RR, Peyrot M, Saudek CD. The effect of a comprehensive diabetes education program incorporating coping skills training on emotional well being and diabetes self efficacy. *Diabetes Educator* 1993; **19**: 210–214.

106. Clement S. Diabetes self-management education. *Diabetes Care* 1995; **1**: 1204–1214.

107. Glasgow RE, Toobert DJ, Hampson SE, Brown JE, Lewinsohn PM, Donnelly J. Improving self-care among older patients with type II diabetes: the 'Sixty Something' study. *Patient Education and Counseling* 1992; **19**: 61–74.

108. Campbell MK, DeVellis BM, Strecher VJ, Ammerman AS. Improving dietary behavior: the effectiveness of tailored messages in primary care settings. *Am J Public Health* 1994; **84**: 783–787.

109. Clark M, Hampson SE, Avery L, Simpson R. Effects of a tailored lifestyle self-management intervention in patients with type 2 diabetes. *Br J Health Psychol* 2004; **9**: 365–379.

110. Bull FC, Kreuter W, Scharff DP. Effects of tailored, personalized and general health messages on physical activity. *Patient Education Counseling* 1999; **36**: 181–192.

111. Glasgow RE, Toobert DJ, Hampson SE. Effects of a brief office-based intervention to facilitate diabetes dietary self-management. *Diabetes Care* 1996; **19**: 835–842.

112. Brug J, De Vries H. Computer-tailored education. In Brug, J, De Vries, H. (eds), special issue. *Patient Education Counseling* 1999; **36**: 99–205.

113. Kayman S, Bruvold W, Stern JS. Maintenance and relapse after weight loss in women: behavioral aspects. *Am J Clin Nutr* 1990; **52**: 800–807.

114. Klem ML, Wing RR, McGuire MI, Seagle HM, Hill JO. A descriptive study of individuals successful at long-term maintenance of substantial weight loss. *Am J Clin Nutr* 1997; **66**: 239–246.

115. Foreyt JP, Goodrick GK. Factors common to successful therapy for the obese patient. *Med Sci Sports Exercise* 1991; **23**: 292–297.

116. Cousins JH, Rubovits DS, Dunn JK, Reeves RS, Ramirez AG, Foreyt JP. Family versus individually oriented intervention for weight loss in Mexican American women. *Public Health Reports* 1992; **107**: 549–555.

117. Sarafino EP, Armstrong JW. *Child and Adolescent Development*, 2nd edn. St. Paul, MN: West, 1986.

118. Zigmond AS, Snaith RP. The Hospital Anxiety and Depression Scale. *Acta Psychiatrica Scandinavica* 1983; **67**: 361–370.

119. Zung WK. A rating instrument for anxiety disorders. *Psychosomatics* 1971; **12**: 371–379.

120. Beck AT, Steer RA, Garbin MG. Psychosomatic properties of the Beck Depression Inventory: twenty-five years of evaluation. *Clin Psychol Rev* 1988; **8**: 77–100.

121. Radloff LS. The CES-D scale: a self-report depression scale for research in the general population. *Appl Psychol Meas* 1977; **1**: 385–401.

122. Wilson W, Ary DV, Biglan A, Glasgow RE, Toobert DJ, Campbell DR. Psychosocial predictors of self-care behaviors (compliance) and glycemic control in non-insulin-dependent diabetes mellitus. *Diabetes Care* 1986; **9**: 614–622.

123. Kavanaugh DJ, Gooley S, Wilson PH. Prediction of adherence and control in diabetes. *J Behav Med* 1993; **16**: 509–522.

124. Skelly AH, Marshall JR, Haughey BP, Davis PJ, Dunford RG. Self-efficacy and confidence in outcomes as determinants of self-care practices in inner-city, African-American women with non-insulin-dependent diabetes. *Diabetes Educator* 1995; **231**: 38–46.

125. Kramer JR, Ledolter J, Manos GN, Bayless ML. Stress and metabolic control in diabetes mellitus: methodological issues and an illustrative analysis. *Ann Behav Med* 2000; **22**: 17–28.

126. Aikens KS, Aikens JE, Wallander JL, Hunt S. Daily activity level buffers stress–glycemia associations in older sedentary NIDDM patients. *J Behav Med* 1997; **20**: 379–390.

127. Surwit RS, Feinglos NN, Scovern AW. Diabetes and behavior: a paradigm for health psychology. *Am Psychol* 1983; **38**: 255–262.

128. Goldston DB, Kovacs M, Obrosky DS, Iyengar S. A longitudinal study of life events and metabolic control among youths with insulin-dependent diabetes mellitus. *Health Psychol* 1995; **14**: 409–414.

129. Kovacs M. Depression in patients with diabetes. *Contemp Intern Med* 1997; **9**: 53–58.

130. Lustman PJ, Anderson RJ, Freedland KE, de Groot M, Carney RM, Clouse RE. Depression and poor glycemic control: a meta-analytic review of the literature. *Diabetes Care* 2000; **23**: 934–942.

131. Talbot F, Nouwen A, Gingras J, Belanger A, Audet J. Relations of diabetes intrusiveness and personal control to symptoms of depression among adults with diabetes. *Health Psychol* 1999; **18**: 537–542.

132. Glasgow RE, McCaul KD, Schafer LC. Barriers to regimen adherence among persons with insulin-dependent diabetes. *J Behav Med* 1986; **9**: 65–77.

133. Polonsky WH, Anderson BJ, Lohrer PA, Aponte JE, Jacobson AM, Cole CF. Insulin omission in women with IDDM. *Diabetes Care* 1994; **17**: 1178–1185.

134. Raymond NR, D'Eramo-Melkus G. Non-insulin-dependent diabetes and obesity in the black and Hispanic population: culturally sensitive management. *Diabetes Educator* 1993; **19**: 313–317.

135. Kilo C, Williamson JR. *Diabetes: the Facts that Let you Regain Control of Your Life.* New York: Wiley, 1987.

136. Parkin T, Skinner TC. Does patient perception of consultation concord with professional perception of consultation. *Diabetes Med* 2002; **19** (Suppl. 2): A14.

137. Clark M, Hampson SE. Comparison of patients and health care professionals beliefs about and attitudes towards type 2 diabetes. *Diabet Med* 2003; **20**: 152–154.

138. Larme AC, Pugh JA. Attitudes of primary care providers toward diabetes. Barriers to guideline implementation. *Diabetes Care* 1998; **21**: 1391–1396.

139. Cerkoney KA, Hart LK. The relationship between the health belief model and compliance of persons with diabetes mellitus. *Diabetes Care* 1980; **3**: 594–598.

140. Polly RK. Diabetes health beliefs, self-care behaviors and glycemic control among older adults with non-insulin dependent diabetes mellitus. *Diabetes Educator* 1992; **18**: 321–327.

141. Hampson SE, Glasgow RE. Dimensional complexity of representations of diabetes and arthritis. *Basic and Applied Social Psychology* 1996; **18**: 45–59.

5

Patient Empowerment

Martha M. Funnell and **Robert M. Anderson**

5.1 Introduction

In 1991, our education team at the University of Michigan Diabetes Research and Training Center (MDRTC) published our first article on patient empowerment. This article offered a new paradigm for diabetes self-management education and care in contrast to the more traditional, medical model approach.[1] This approach grew out of the frustration that we along with others felt with our existing health care systems that were designed to care for the acutely ill and were not prepared to effectively care for chronic illnesses such as diabetes. Health care professionals struggled to give the recommended levels of diabetes care within the constraints of a busy office practice. We also struggled with the reality of dealing with a chronic illness where the outcomes are largely dependent on the patients' self-care behaviours.

Diabetes care is radically different from the treatment of acute illness and therefore requires a different conceptual framework to inform the behavioral, educational and clinical approaches used to treat it.[2–4] Traditionally, the success of patients and health professionals has been judged by the ability of patients to successfully adhere or comply with their treatment plan. A great deal of effort has been spent to try to both measure and increase adherence or compliance. Unfortunately, this paradigm does not match the reality of a chronic illness such as diabetes.

Empowerment, on the other hand, recognizes that people with diabetes are fully responsible for the self-management of their illness. This responsibility is non-negotiable and inescapable. When we adopt this paradigm, we redefine the roles and responsibilities of patients and health professionals and implement a patient-centred approach to diabetes care.

Psychology in Diabetes Care   Edited by Frank J. Snoek and T. Chas Skinner
© 2005 John Wiley & Sons, Ltd.

5.2 Empowerment Defined

Empowerment is defined as helping patients discover and develop their inherent capacity to be responsible for their own lives and gain mastery over their diabetes.[1] This responsibility is present because of three characteristics of the disease. First, the most important choices affecting the health and well-being of a person with diabetes are made by the person with the disease, not by diabetes educators or physicians. The choices that patients make about eating, physical activity, stress management, monitoring etc. are the major determinants of their diabetes control. Each day, during the routine conduct of their lives, patients with diabetes make a series of choices that, cumulatively, have a far greater impact on their blood glucose levels, quality of life and overall health and well-being than the decisions made by the health professionals providing their care. Although health professionals are experts on diabetes, patients are experts on their own lives and what will work best for them.

Second, patients are in control of their diabetes self-management. No matter what health professionals do or say, patients are in control of the important daily diabetes self-management decisions. We may advise, educate, plead, persuade, cajole or encourage, but when patients leave the clinic they have control over their self-management choices. Patients can choose to accept or reject any recommendation made by a health professional, no matter how important or relevant the health care professional believes that recommendation to be.

Third, the consequences of the choices patients make every day about their diabetes care accrue first and foremost to patients. Health professionals cannot share in the risk of developing complications of diabetes, nor can they share in the cost to the patient's quality of life of making a commitment to rigorous blood glucose control. Diabetes belongs to the patient. Knowing what is best for a patient's diabetes is not the same as knowing what is best for that person.

Most of the training health professionals receive is based on the treatment of acute illnesses where professionals are socialized to accept responsibility to treat or solve problems that patients cannot manage on their own. Most health professionals feel this responsibility very deeply. It happens almost every time they interact with their patients. This sense of responsibility also influences how they define their effectiveness. Health professionals usually feel effective when they are able to come up with therapies and solutions to their patients' health care problems and frustrated when they cannot. In an illness such as diabetes where the patient's self-management decisions determine the outcome, conflict and frustration often result.

This is particularly true when the plan focuses solely on the physical aspects of the patient's diabetes and has not taken into account the patient's psychological health and well-being, goals, culture and lifestyle. Health professionals, grounded in the traditional medical model, often feel that it is their responsibility to get their patients to maximize their level of glucose control in order to prevent the acute and chronic complications of diabetes. Furthermore, they usually view education as a process to accomplish this goal. However, since they cannot control the patient's behaviour in order to reach the goal, they are likely to feel dissatisfied with diabetes self-management education and care. Because our view of success is shaped by the acute care paradigm, patients are often labelled 'non-compliant' as an expression of our frustration in our inability to solve their problems.

Patients also express dissatisfaction with being seen as just an A1C number and not having their goals, struggles and hard work acknowledged by health care professionals. The end result is that diabetes care is less than optimal and patients suffer needlessly from its devastating complications.

Empowerment on the other hand grows out of the traditions of community psychology,[5] adult education[6] and counselling psychology[7] that view the purpose of education as enabling the recipients to gain more power over their lives, increase the number of choices available to them and enhance their ability to influence the individuals and organizations that affect their lives. Empowerment emphasizes the whole person and embraces a biopsychosocial model of disease and illness, as opposed to the more hierarchical, biological reductionist and compliance-oriented models derived from the treatment of acute illnesses.[8]

In the empowerment approach, diabetes self-management education is viewed as 'a collaboration among equals' designed to help patients make informed decisions about their own diabetes self-management. The knowledge necessary to make informed decisions about diabetes care falls into two global domains.[9] The first domain is knowledge about diabetes and its treatment, i.e. the information necessary to make cost–benefit judgments about adopting (or not adopting) various diabetes self-management options. The second domain is self-awareness about the patient's own needs, values, goals and aspirations regarding diabetes care. In education directed at this latter domain, patients are helped to examine and clarify the emotional, social, intellectual and spiritual components of their lives as they relate to the decisions they must make about their diabetes self-management. Diabetes care is then incorporated into the patient's life, rather than the reverse.

5.3 Patient Empowerment and Diabetes

Patient empowerment was first noted in the diabetes literature in 1991.[1] Since that time, this paradigm has been tested by us and others both in practice and in controlled trials and has been increasingly recognized as both an efficacious and practical approach to diabetes self-management education and care.[10] While many factors support changes in health care, which in turn affect other changes, there are multiple examples of the influence of the philosophy of empowerment on diabetes since 1991. These include increased emphasis on collaboration with patients,[11–15] patient-centred care as part of chronic disease management,[11–14, 16–21] collaborative goal-setting,[12,14,16,21,22] theoretically based, integrated educational strategies, increased emphasis on self-management skills[21–28] and psychosocial issues[29–32] and a decreased emphasis on compliance and adherence,[2–4] information transfer[12,23–26] and didactic presentations.[12,21,23–26] There has also been global acknowledgement of this approach in multiple countries as part of standards for diabetes self-management education and care.

A number of studies have documented the effectiveness of the empowerment approach and use of compatible strategies (e.g. collaborative care, problem-based education).[11,12,14,15,17,19,20] Patients do set goals and achieve outcomes that are personally and clinically meaningful, even when not directed to do so.[33] Because these goals are meaningful for them and chosen by them, they are more likely to be attained and sustained than those imposed by health care professionals.

5.4   Implementing the Empowerment Approach

In order to manage diabetes successfully, patients need to be able to set goals, and make decisions that are effective and fit with their lifestyles, while taking into account many metabolic, psychosocial and personal factors.[34] Intervention strategies that enable patients to make informed decisions about goals, treatment options and self-care behaviours and assume responsibility for their daily diabetes management are effective in helping patients to care for themselves. In order to effectively implement this approach, patients need education designed to promote informed decision-making and professionals need to educate and provide on-going support for patients' self-management efforts and practice in ways that are consistent with this philosophy.

5.5   Implementing the Empowerment Approach in Diabetes Self-Management Education (DSME)

Diabetes self-management education (DSME) is the essential first step in patient empowerment. Patients need to be able to care for themselves safely and effectively and to understand the consequences of their decisions. Without DSME patients cannot make or implement informed self-management decisions. The empowerment approach to DSME seeks to maximize the self-management knowledge, skills, self-awareness and sense of personal autonomy to enable patients to take charge of their own diabetes care. Empowered patients are those who have learned enough about diabetes and themselves, so that they can select and achieve their own goals for diabetes care.[1]

Empowerment-based DSME can be provided in both individual and group teaching sessions. Much of the clinical content provided within this approach is the same as in a traditional diabetes education programme. In addition, patients need information about various therapeutic options, the negatives and positives for each of these options, how to make behaviour changes, how to solve problems and how to cope with the psychosocial demands of living with a chronic illness. They also need to understand their role as decision-makers and the responsibility they have for self-care and ultimately for their own outcomes.

While many of the teaching methods, tools or strategies are similar to those in other approaches, their purpose and use is often different. For example, goal setting is used to help patients identify and attain their own self-care goals. This is in contrast to negotiating metabolic and other goals that we choose for patients and then using their achievement of those goals as a way to judge their self-care ability and level of compliance.

People with diabetes do not experience diabetes in discreet categories – they experience its impact on their lives holistically. Educational methods within the empowerment model incorporate interactive teaching strategies designed to integrate the clinical with the behavioural and psychosocial aspects of self-care, involve patients in problem solving and address their psychosocial and cultural needs. Using patient experiences as the curriculum helps to individualize group educational programmes and ensure that the content is relevant for the participants.

Strategies for implementing this approach range from simply assessing needs (e.g. Do you have cultural or religious beliefs and practices that influence how you care for your diabetes?) to a discussion of roles and responsibilities, incorporating the totality of diabetes care into a discussion, to providing an entire education programme based on patient experiences and problems.

As an example of a strategy to help patients integrate clinical information with their experiences, an educator might incorporate the following questions during a discussion on how to perform self-blood glucose monitoring (SBGM) and interpret and use the results:

- How often do you need to test in order to manage your diabetes?

- How will you remember to test at home? Away from home?

- Do you want your family and friends to remind you to test? Ask about the results?

- How will you test in public places? How will you respond if others ask what you are doing?

- How will you feel if the results are not what you expected or hoped? How will you respond? How will this affect your self-care?

Using the patients' experiences and problems as the curriculum for a group diabetes self-management education programme is another effective strategy within the framework of empowerment. Providing individual patients with their test results and encouraging them to conduct self-management experiments between sessions can be used to create a problem-based curriculum.

As one example, in a recent six-session group programme offered weekly to African American patients,[35] clinical content was presented in response to issues or questions raised by patients. No pre-determined lectures were given. At the end of each of the six sessions, those who wished chose a short-term goal as a self-management experiment to try that week. We began each subsequent session with a discussion of what was learned from the experiment. These experiences and other problems and questions raised by the group were then used to discuss diabetes content and self-management, psychosocial issues and other concerns. Although strategies for implementation varied, there were five components that were part of each session that served as the structure for this programme.[36] These include

- reflecting on relevant experiences

- discussing the role of emotion

- engaging in systematic goal-setting and problem-solving

- answering clinical questions

- providing feedback to instructors about the session.

Table 5.1 provides an assessment instrument designed to determine whether the DSME programme is in keeping with the empowerment philosophy. The evaluation of a DSME programme based on the empowerment approach also needs to include patient achievement of self-selected diabetes care goals, improved psychosocial adaptation and enhanced self-efficacy, along with metabolic control. An additional measure of success is the relationship that the educator and patients create based on a true partnership where both the expertise of the patient and the professional are equally valued.

Table 5.1 Empowerment-based DSME programme assessment

How much does your program *explicitly*
  Affirm that the person with diabetes is responsible for, and in control of the daily self-management of diabetes?
  Educate participants in ways that promote informed decision-making, rather than trying to influence adherence/compliance?
  Teach participants to set behavioural goals so that they can make changes of their own choosing?
  Integrate clinical, psychosocial and behavioural aspects of diabetes self-management?
  Affirm that the participants are experts on their own learning needs?
  Affirm the ability of participants to determine an approach to diabetes self-management that will work for them?
  Affirm the innate capacity of patients to identify and learn to solve their own problems?
  Respect the cultural, ethnic and religious beliefs of the target population?
  Create opportunities for social support?
  Provide on-going self-management support?

5.6 Implementing the Empowerment Approach in Diabetes Self-Management Support (DSMS)

Diabetes self-management education has generally been shown to be effective for improving metabolic and psychosocial outcomes in the short term;[24,25,27] however, a one-time educational programme rarely succeeds in helping patients sustain the types of behaviour needed for successful diabetes self-care. They also need on-going self-management support (DSMS) to continue to address educational, psychosocial and behavioural needs. Like DSME, empowerment-based DSMS can be provided in both individual and group sessions.

Goal-setting is an effective strategy to provide on-going DSMS. Table 5.2 outlines goal-setting as defined by the empowerment approach.[37,38] We use a

Table 5.2 Behaviour change protocol. Copyright © 2004 American Diabetes Association. From Clinical Diabetes, Vol. 22, 004: 123–127. Reprinted with permission from The American Diabetes Association

---

Step I: explore the problem or issue (past)

- What is the hardest thing about caring for diabetes for you?
- Please tell me more about that.
- Are there some specific examples you can give me?

Step II: clarify feelings and meaning (present)

- What are your thoughts about this?
- Are you feeling [insert feeling] because [insert meaning]?

Step III: develop a plan (future)

- What do you want?
- How would this situation have to change for you to feel better about it?
- Where would you like to be regarding this situation in (specific time, e.g. 1 month, 3 months, 1 year)?
- What are your options?
- What are barriers for you?
- Who could help you?
- What are the costs and benefits for each of your choices?
- What would happen if you do not do anything about it?
- How important is it, on a scale of 1 to 10, for you to do something about this?
- Let's develop a plan.

Step IV: commit to action (future)

- Are you willing to do what you need to do to solve this problem?
- What are some steps you could take?
- What are you going to do?
- When are you going to do it?
- How will you know if you have succeeded?
- What is one thing you will do when you leave here today?

Step V: experience and evaluate the plan (future)

- How did it go?
- What did you learn?
- What barriers did you encounter?
- What, if anything, would you do differently next time?
- What will you do when you leave here today?

---

five-step process to provide patients with the understanding, clarity and experience of setting and achieving their self-selected behavioural goals. The first two steps define the problem and associated thoughts and feelings that can help or hinder goal attainment. The third step is to identify the long term goal and the fourth the specific behavioural action step the patient will take towards achievement of the long term goal. After patients carry out a self-management experiment, they are helped to determine what was learned and identify the next self-management step. The process then begins again.

Patients are encouraged to think of these steps as self-management experiments rather than as successes or failures. Reflecting on their experiments leads to learning that can then be used to guide the next step in the process. Each experiment provides information about the true nature of the problem, barriers and available supports and effective next steps. The role of the professional is to actively listen and help the patient to obtain clarity about diabetes self-care problems, feelings and goals, collaborate and provide information and offer support and outside resources.

5.7 Implementing the Empowerment Approach in Diabetes Care

Once health professionals embrace the empowerment philosophy their relationships with patients and the structure and process of their practices also change to better support their patients' empowerment and attainment of self-selected diabetes care goals. Table 5.3 outlines individual and practice redesign strategies that can be used to support patient empowerment.

The roles that health professionals and patients have traditionally assumed also change in this philosophy. The paternalistic approach traditionally assumed by physicians, and the maternalistic approach traditionally assumed by nurses and educators, is not effective for a self-managed illness. Rather than a parent–child relationship, a partnership needs to be established. Table 5.4 outlines the roles and responsibilities of both patients and health care professionals.[39] Because this is often a new role for patients, it is helpful to have a discussion early in the diabetes care process about the responsibilities that we each have. For example, we usually begin by noting that while as professionals we are experts in diabetes, we are not experts on that patient's life. It takes both knowledge of diabetes and knowledge of what will work well for that individual to create an effective diabetes care plan, which takes a shared expertise. It is also helpful to point out that it may take several attempts to create the right plan. If the plan does not work at first, it does not mean that either the patient or the health professional is not doing a good job. It just means that a new plan is needed. We also let patients know that we understand the difficulties of living with diabetes and that we are there to help and support and offer information about available resources.

Table 5.3 Health professional and practice-based strategies to support patient empowerment. Copyright © 2004 American Diabetes Association. From therapy for Diabertes Related Disorders, 4th Edition. Reprinted with permission from The American Diabetes Association

Health professional strategies

- Stress the seriousness of diabetes.
- Stress the importance of DSME and DSMS.
- Stress the importance of the patient's role in self-management.
- Offer referral to a DSME programme, diabetes educator, dietitian and mental health professionals as needed.
- Reinforce education provided in the DSME programme.
- Begin each visit with an assessment of the patient's concerns, questions and progress towards metabolic and behavioural goals.
- Address patient identified fears and concerns.
- Assess patients' opinions about home blood glucose monitoring results and other laboratory and outcome measures.
- Review and revise the diabetes care plan as needed based on both the patients' and health care professionals' assessment of its effectiveness.
- Provide on-going information about the costs and benefits of therapeutic and behavioural options.
- Take advantage of teachable moments that occur during each visit.
- Establish a partnership with patients and their families.
- Provide information about behaviour change and problem solving strategies.
- Assist patients to solve problems and overcome barriers to self-management.
- Support and facilitate patients in their role as self-management decision-makers.
- Abandon traditional dysfunctional models of care (e.g. adherence, compliance).

Practice-based strategies

- Link patient self-management support with health care professional support (e.g. system changes, patient flow, logistics).
- Supplement DSMS with information technology.
- Incorporate DSMS into practical interventions, coordinated by nurse case managers or other staff members.
- Create a team with other health care professionals in your system or area with additional experience or training in the clinical, educational and behavioural or psychosocial aspects of diabetes care.
- Replace individual visits with group or cluster visits to provide efficient and effective self-management support.
- Assist patients to select one area of self-management on which to concentrate that can be reinforced by all team members.
- Create a patient-centred environment that incorporates self-management support from all practice personnel and is integrated into the flow of the visit.

As professionals we also need to listen more to our patients and offer less advice.[40] Asking questions and using reflective listening techniques can help patients reflect on issues or problems and lead to the identification of effective strategies.[41] We can also show that we care about our patients as individuals first and not just about their diabetes or blood glucose. Rather than beginning each visit with a review of the patient's glucose log, asking how they are feeling, about progress towards goals, their thoughts about how they perceive their diabetes is

Table 5.4   Roles and responsibilities of patients and health care professionals. Reproduced from Funell, Anderson, Current Diabetes Reports 2003; 3 128, with permission of Current Science Inc., Philadelphia

Health care professionals

- Provide information so that patients can make informed decisions about the costs and benefits of therapeutic and behavioural options
- Create a patient-centred environment
- Establish a partnership with patients and their families
- Provide information about behaviour change and problem-solving strategies
- Develop collaborative goals
- Support and facilitate patients in their role as self-management decision-makers
- Abandon traditional dysfunctional models of care (e.g. adherence, compliance)

Patients with diabetes

- Provide information about feelings, values, needs and abilities
- Establish a partnership with health care team
- Assume responsibility for diabetes self-management decision-making and outcomes
- Develop and work toward self-selected goals
- Become an active, knowledgeable consumer of diabetes care

currently managed and what they would like to accomplish during the visit can lead to highly productive discussions that take no more time than a traditional appointment.

5.8   Costs and Benefits of the Empowerment Approach

There are both challenges and benefits for adopting and implementing this approach. For some it can be difficult to give up their traditional roles and responsibilities. As professionals, we have long had the illusion that we are in control of our patients' diabetes self-management. The empowerment philosophy requires that we acknowledge the control that patients have over their decisions, lives and outcomes. It also means that we need to see our patients in a new light, acknowledge their equality in our relationship with them and interact as partners, rather than as parents and children. We become responsible to our patients rather than for our patients.

Setting goals with rather than for patients can also be difficult. It is hard when patients choose goals that do not seem meaningful to us as health professionals. Adopting the empowerment philosophy implies that we trust patients' ability to make wise decisions and set goals that are meaningful in the context of their lives, not just their diabetes care. Our responsibility is to provide the information on which they can base those decisions.

Another concern is the amount of time that will be spent if we listen, set goals or address the patient's concerns before our own. It has been our experience that this increases the efficiency of the visit and ultimately decreases the amount of time spent. Starting a visit with statements such as 'What is important for us to accomplish in the 15 minutes that we have today?' or using a short form to be completed by the patient while waiting to identify key needs and questions can help to streamline and focus the visit.

Some patients also struggle with this approach. They may feel overwhelmed or are not able to take on this level of responsibility. They may tell us that they just want to be told what to do. In those situations, we acknowledge that they have given us the responsibility for making those decisions. We also let them know that if they get tired of the plan we have created for them, to let us know and we will work together to change it. It is also important not to assume that patients who are newly diagnosed, elderly or have other health issues are necessarily part of this group without their explicitly letting us know that they are giving these decisions back to us.

It can also be difficult to address negative emotional issues that patients may raise related to diabetes or its treatment or other aspects of their lives. As health professionals, our tendency is to try to minimize or ignore these concerns and their effects. However, these strategies rarely work for any length of time. In addition, patients may continue to raise these concerns and actually lengthen the visit.[41]

There are also many benefits to this approach. One of the greatest benefits is the type of relationship that we can create with our patients. We are able to be supportive and helpful in ways that we were not in the more traditional model. As we eliminate attempting to do the impossible (e.g. motivate or get other people to change) our own frustration decreases. Once we know that we are no longer responsible to solve patients' emotional and behavioural problems, we are able to listen and respond empathetically rather than trying to think of a solution. We are then able to focus on the patient as a person and not just on their diabetes.

The ultimate benefit is that it works. Patients do achieve positive metabolic and other positive outcomes. We have seen both improvements in laboratory values and in quality of life. As health professionals, we also experience benefits in terms of decreased frustration and less burn-out. We are able to work effectively with our patients and become true partners in their journey with diabetes.

5.9 Concluding Thoughts

This chapter has summarized the processes that led us to rethink and redefine diabetes self-management education and care. We have described progress in the adoption and implementation of this philosophy over the last decade. We have highlighted the research, both our own and that of our colleagues, that we feel provides evidence for the effectiveness of this approach. We are convinced, on philosophical, theoretical, experiential and evidential grounds, that this approach is effective and that additional models need to be developed and tested in a variety of health care systems throughout the world.

Acknowledgment

Work on this chapter was supported in part by grant numbers NIH5P60 DK20572 and 1 R18 0K062323 from the National Institute of Diabetes and Digestive and Kidney Diseases of the National Institutes of Health.

References

1. Funnell MM, Anderson RM, Arnold MS, Barr PA, Donnelly MB, Johnson PD, Taylor-Moon D, White NH. Empowerment: an idea whose time has come in diabetes patient education. *Diabetes Educ* 1991; **17**: 37–41.
2. Funnell MM, Anderson RM. The problem with compliance in diabetes. *JAMA* 2000; **284**: 1709.
3. Anderson RM, Funnell MM. Compliance and adherence are dysfunctional concepts in diabetes care. *Diabetes Educ* 2000; **26**: 597–604.
4. Glasgow RE, Anderson RM. In diabetes care moving from compliance to adherence is not enough. *Diabetes Care* 1999; **22**: 2090–2091.
5. Rapport J. Terms of empowerment exemplars of prevention: toward a theory for community psychology. *Am J Community Psychol* 1987; **14**: 12–47.
6. Wallerstein N, Bernstein E. Empowerment education: Freir's ideas adapted to health education. *Health Education Q* 1988; **15**: 379–394.
7. Combs AW, Avila DL, Purkey WW. *Helping Relationships*, 2nd edn. Boston, MA: Allyn and Bacon, 1978.
8. Engel GL. The need for a new medical model: a challenge for biomedicine. *Science* 1977; **196**: 129–136.
9. Anderson RM, Funnell MM, Barr PA, Dedrick RF, Davis WK. Learning to empower patients: the results of a professional education program for diabetes educators. *Diabetes Care* 1991; **14**: 584–590.
10. Funnell MM, Anderson RM. Patient empowerment: a look back, a look ahead. *Diabetes Educ* 2003; **29**: 454–464.
11. Von Korff M, Gruman J, Schaefer J, Curry SJ, Wagner EH. Collaborative management of chronic illness. *Ann Intern Med* 1997; **127**: 1097–1102.
12. Piette JD, Glasgow RE. Strategies for improving behavioural and health outcomes among patients with diabetes: self-management education. In Gerstein HC, Haynes RB (eds), *Evidence-Based Diabetes Care*. Ontario, CA: Decker, 2001, pp 207–251.
13. Glasgow RE, Hiss RG, Anderson RM, Friedman NM, Hayward RA, Marrero DG, Taylor CB, Vinicor F. Report of the health care delivery work group. *Diabetes Care* 2001; **24**: 124–130.
14. Glasgow RE, Funnell MM, Bonomi AE, Davis CL, Beckham V, Wagner EH. Self-management aspects of the Improving Chronic Illness Care Breakthrough series: design and implementation with diabetes and heart failure teams. *Ann Behav Med* 2002; **24**: 80–87.
15. Williams GC, Zeldman A. Patient-centered diabetes self-management education. *Current Med* 2002; **2**: 145–152.
16. Glasgow RE, Eakins EG. Medical office-based interventions. In: FJ Snoek, TC Skinner (eds), *Psychology in Diabetes Care*. Chichester: Wiley, 2000; pp 141–168.
17. Hiss RG, Gillard ML, Armbruster BA, McClure LA. Comprehensive evaluation of community-based diabetic patients: effect of feedback to patients and their physicians: a randomized controlled trial. *Diabetes Care* 2001; **24**: 690–694.

18. Wagner EH, Glasgow RE, David C, Bonomi AE, Provost L, McCulloch D, Carver P, Sixta C. Quality improvement in chronic illness care: a collaborative approach. *Joint Commission J Quality Improvement* 2001; **27**: 63–80.
19. Renders CM, Valk GD, Griffin S, Wagner EH, Eijk JT, Assendelft WJ. Interventions to improve the management of diabetes mellitus in primary care, outpatient and community settings. *Cochrane Database Systematic Rev* 2001; **1**: CD001481.
20. Wagner EH, Grothaus LC, Sandhu N, Galvin MS, McGregor M, Artz K, Coleman EA. Chronic care clinics for diabetes in primary care: a system-wide randomized trial. *Diabetes Care* 2001; **24**: 695–700.
21. Funnell MM, Anderson RM. Changing office practice and health care systems to facilitate diabetes self-management. *Current Diabetes Rep* 2003; **3**: 127–133.
22. Mensing C, Boucher J, Cypress M, Weinger K, Barta P, Hosey G, Kopher W, Lasichak A, Lamb B, Mangan M, Norman J, Tanja J, Yauk L, Wisdom K, Adams C. National standards for diabetes self-management education. *Diabetes Care* 2000; **23**: 682–689.
23. Roter DL, Hall JA, Merisca R, Nordstrom B, Cretin D, Svarstad B. Effectiveness of interventions to improve patient compliance: a meta-analysis. *Med Care* 1998; **36**: 1138–1161.
24. Norris SL, Engelgau MM, Naranyan KMV. Effectiveness of self-management training in type 2 diabetes: a systematic review of randomized controlled trials. *Diabetes Care* 2001; **24**: 561–587.
25. Norris SL, Lau J, Smith SJ, Schmid CH, Engelgau MM. Self-management education for adults with type 2 diabetes: a meta-analysis on the effect on glycemic control. *Diabetes Care* 2002; **25**: 1159–1171.
26. Barlow J, Wright C, Sheasby J, Turner A, Hainsworth J. Self-management approaches for people with chronic condition: a review. *Patient Education Counselling* 2002; **48**: 177–187.
27. Brown SA. Interventions to promote diabetes self-management: state of the science. *Diabetes Educ* 1999; **25** (Suppl.): 52–61.
28. Funnell MM, Anderson RM. Putting Humpty Dumpty back together again: reintegrating the clinical and behavioural components in diabetes care and education. *Diabetes Spectrum* 1999; **12**: 19–23.
29. Rubin RR. Facilitating self-care in people with diabetes. *Diabetes Spectrum* 2001; **14**: 55–57.
30. Lustman PJ, Anderson RJ, Freedland KE, DeGroot M, Carney RM, Clouse RE. Depression and poor glucose control: a review of the literature. *Diabetes Care* 2000; **23**: 934–942.
31. Polonsky WH. Listening to our patients' concerns: understanding and addressing diabetes-specific emotional distress. *Diabetes Spectrum* 1996; **9**: 8–11.
32. Testa MA, Simonson DC. Health economic benefits and quality of life during improved glycemic control in patients with type 2 diabetes mellitus: a randomized, controlled, double-blind trial. *JAMA* 1998; **280**: 1490–1496.
33. Anderson RM, Funnell MM, Butler PM, Arnold MS, Feste CC. Patient empowerment: results of a randomized controlled trial. *Diabetes Care* 1995; **18**: 943–949.
34. Funnell MM, Anderson RM. Empowerment and self-management education. *Clinical Diabetes* 2004; **22**: 123–127.
35. Anderson RM, Funnell MM, Nwankwo R, Gillard ML, Oh M, Fitzgerald TJ. Evaluating a problem-based empowerment program for African Americans with diabetes: results of a randomized controlled trial. *Ethnicity and Disease*, 2nd edn 2005.
36. Funnell MM, Nwankwo R, Gillard ML, Anderson RM, Tang TS. Implementing an empowerment-based diabetes self-management education program. *Diabetes Educ* 2005; **31**: 53–61.
37. Anderson RM, Funnell MM. *The Art of Empowerment: Stories and Strategies for Diabetes Educators*. Alexandria, VA: American Diabetes Association, 2000.

38. Anderson RM, Funnell MM, Arnold MS. Using the empowerment approach to help patient change behaviour. In Anderson BJ, Rubin RR (eds), *Practical Psychology for Diabetes Clinicians*, 2nd edn. Alexandria, VA: American Diabetes Association, 2002, pp 3–12.

39. Funnell MM, Anderson RM. Role of diabetes education in patient management. In Lebovitz H (ed.), *Therapy for Diabetes Mellitus and Related Disorders*, 4th edn. Alexandria, VA: American Diabetes Association, 2004, pp 106–111.

40. Marvel MK, Epstein RM, Flowers K, Beckman HB. Soliciting the patient's agenda: have we improved? *JAMA* 1999; **281**: 283–287.

41. Levinson W, Gorawara-Bhat R, Lamb J. A study of patient clues and physician responses in primary care and surgical settings. *JAMA* 2000; **284**: 1021–1027.

6

Medical Office-Based Interventions

Russell E. Glasgow

6.1 Theoretical Background

When one thinks of psychologists in diabetes, the image that comes to mind is that of a patient discussing emotional difficulties with a therapist in a mental health setting. This stereotype, based on a referral system for behavioural health care, was generally accurate for many years. Today, however, the role of psychology and behavioural science in diabetes is changing, spurred by new evidence, the development of brief behavioural interventions and the information technology revolution.[1-4]

Both the range of issues addressed by psychology and the modalities of intervention have expanded significantly. Psychologists and other health professionals are increasingly involved in diabetes care. In some instances, they are part of multidisciplinary teams that provide direct patient care in medical offices. In other cases, they supervise practice innovations, design computer-assisted intervention programs or instruct other health professionals in behaviour change or organizational change principles and strategies.

There is an important need for psychologists to be more involved in the diabetes care that takes place in medical offices for three primary reasons. First, many patients will not or cannot avail themselves of psychological assistance offered via the traditional referral system. Patients frequently have many barriers to following through on referrals, including cost, lack of familiarity with behavioural science, inconvenience, the time commitment required and anticipated stigma associated with 'seeing a shrink'. Second, the quality of care provided for diabetes patients in most medical settings is substantially suboptimal.[5-7] Almost all population-based

Psychology in Diabetes Care   Edited by Frank J. Snoek and T. Chas Skinner
© 2005 John Wiley & Sons, Ltd.

studies of the level of recommended 'best practices' received by patients have revealed much lower than desired rates of screening and clinical services.[5,6] The rates of preventive services and especially lifestyle change interventions are even lower.[6–8] Third, patient-centred, motivational interviewing and patient activation/empowerment approaches have been found to produce beneficial effects, yet such strategies are seldom employed in either primary care or specialty endocrinological settings. Thus, there is a compelling need and great opportunity to apply behavioural science in medical office settings.

From a conceptual and social–environmental influence perspective,[9,10] the medical office setting occupies a strategic position in the 'pyramid of social–environmental' influences on patient self-management and decision-making processes (Figure 6.1). As can be seen in this figure, health care system encounters fall midway between the more proximal influences such as personal actions and family and friends on one hand and more distal factors such as community and media/policy influences on the other. Because of this position and the enormous credibility accorded physicians and other health care professionals in our society, interventions in medical settings have great potential to also leverage the other levels of social–environmental factors.

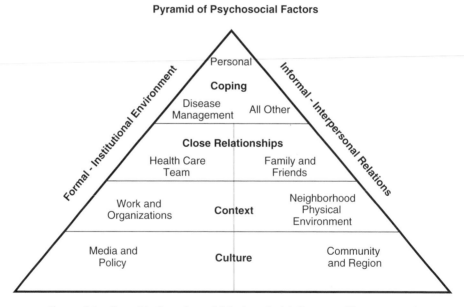

Figure 6.1   Pyramid of psychosocial factors that influence self-management

The medical office setting also has much to recommend it due to the frequent contact most diabetes patients have with their health care providers. On average, patients with diabetes see their doctor for several visits per year. This repeated, ongoing contact provides a potent context within which to work with patients to collaboratively set goals, develop strategies, collect information, provide feedback and modify goals or set new ones.[1,11,12] Another important asset from a public health perspective is the availability of medical records, and the increasing prevalence of diabetes registries, which permit population-based disease management activities.[13]

To take advantage of these opportunities, however, many psychologists will have to change how they do business.[1] In particular, they will need to adapt their assessment and intervention strategies to be compatible with and to fit into medical settings. In addition, they need to understand the world views and training of physicians (as well as nurses, dietitians, health educators and other health care professionals) and how these frequently differ from those to which psychologists have been acculturated in their own training and practice.

6.2   Clinical and Logistical Rationale
   for Office-Based Intervention

As noted above, the majority of patients with diabetes do not attend psychosocial disease management programmes, nor do most attend traditional diabetes education programmes.[14,15] Thus, we must look for other avenues via which to deliver behavioural interventions. The physician office visit is one such avenue, as most patients with diabetes (with access to health care) make frequent, often quarterly, visits to a health care provider. Even in the context of a brief office visit, the physician has a key role in helping the patient to better manage his or her diabetes,[16–18] since the physician is seen as the expert. Anderson and Funnell[17] describe the office visit as a 'teachable moment', a time when patients are very motivated to listen to and act on the advice of the physician (and other health care team members). This is especially true if the visit represents something novel for the patient; for example, if the patient is newly diagnosed, beginning to experience chronic complications, started on insulin or referred to an endocrinologist for expert consultation. Thus, the physician office visit provides an opportunity to reach the majority of patients with diabetes and to do so with a highly credible source of information. Providers are often overwhelmed by multiple demands and time pressures,[19,20] and are reluctant to add yet another protocol into the busy office setting. In addition, studies of physician barriers to delivering behavioural interventions indicate that many physicians feel ill equipped to counsel patients regarding behaviour change.[2,21] Commonly reported physician barriers include lack of training in behavioural counselling, lack of time, lack of reimbursement for such counselling and doubts as to the efficacy of such interventions.

Tremendous opportunities for behavioural science contributions exist, given the complexity of the biopsychosocial issues in diabetes, the frequency of contact with diabetes patients and the relatively low level of adherence to recommended guidelines[22-25] by both patients and providers.[6,26] To impact diabetes management, behavioural and psychological assessments, interventions and models should be practical and efficient, readily understood by non-psychologists and address issues diabetes patients and providers (rather than psychologists) perceive as important.[27-29] Behavioural assessments and interventions must also be brief and integrated into the regular clinic flow. The use of interactive computer-based health care technology[4,30,31] that collects and immediately scores key behavioural assessment information and delivers, in full or in part, behavioural interventions addresses this issue. Other ways to achieve this goal involve transferring management responsibilities to non-physician (and probably non-mental-health professional) members of the health care team such as nurses, dietitians or diabetes educators. Specific suggestions for incorporating brief, behavioural assessments and interventions into primary care settings are discussed in section 6.5.

6.3   Research Findings from Office-Based Interventions

There are at least three types of psychosocial research directly related to medical office practices, as well as a much broader array of psychosocial assessment and treatment activities such as referral to lifestyle behaviour change, programmes such as the Diabetes Prevention Program,[32] or mental health services reviewed elsewhere. These types of research are (a) psychosocial interventions conducted during the course of regular office visits, (b) system interventions to alter the health care setting and (c) training interventions to change the behaviour of physicians, nurses or other health professionals. A brief summary of key illustrative research is provided for each of these topics.

I also describe briefly relevant medical office applications conducted with other chronic illnesses to illustrate opportunities in cases where similar research in diabetes has not yet been conducted. First, however, let me describe the framework that will be used to evaluate the extant literature. Termed the RE-AIM model, this framework focuses attention on important applicability issues and a real world, effectiveness perspective[29,33,34] compatible with the realities of medical office treatment of diabetes at the beginning of the 21st century. There are five component dimensions to the RE-AIM model, which combine to determine the overall public health impact of an intervention: (1) *reach*, or the percentage and representativeness of patients who are willing to participate in a given procedure; (2) *efficacy*, or the impact of an intervention on important outcomes, including behavioural, biologic, quality of life (and any negative outcomes) and economic outcomes. There are also three less often studied, but equally important outcomes, which concern impact at the level of a medical office or health care system. These 'AIM' dimensions are (3) *adoption*, or the percentage and representativeness of settings and clinical staff that are willing to adopt or try an office innovation; (4) *implementation*, or how consistently a protocol is delivered as intended, and (5)

maintenance, or the extent to which a programme or policy becomes institutionalized or part of the routine practice of medical settings. These five factors each
represent different aspects of the public health impact of a programme. Several
reviews have documented that the setting level or 'AIM' dimensions of the RE-
AIM framework, which are just as important as the individual level dimensions,
are seldom reported.[35,36]

An example may help to illustrate how the RE-AIM evaluation framework can
lead to surprising conclusions about the wisest use of scarce health care resources.
The overall public health impact of an intervention is an interaction among these
factors which can be represented as a multiplicative relationship. Therefore, an
intervention that is highly efficacious – say .7 – (see Table 6.1) (such as intensive
group self-management education), but has very limited reach or appeal (.1), may
prove to have little overall impact ($.7 \times .1 = .07$) and less population-wide benefit
than a more modest intervention that has less efficacy (.3) but higher reach
$(.5)(.3 \times .5 = .15)$.

Table 6.1 Component dimensions and related characteristics of the RE-AIM evaluation
framework

Evaluation Dimension	Units and level of measurement	Amount of research
% **Reach** (what proportion of the panel of patients will receive or be willing and able to participate in this intervention?)	Percentage and representativeness of members of a population that participate	Modest
% **Efficacy** (success rates if implemented as in guidelines: defined as positive outcomes minus negative outcomes)	Magnitude or percentage of improvement on outcome(s) of interest	Substantial
% **Adoption** (how many settings, practices and plans will adopt this intervention?)	Percentage and representativeness of organizations and clinicians that try an intervention	Minimal
% **Implementation** (to what extent is the intervention implemented as intended in the real world?)	Consistency and quality of intervention delivery under real-world conditions	Moderate
% **Maintenance** (extent to which a programme is sustained over time)	Extent to which individuals or implementation agents continue to deliver a programme over time	Minimal

This way of thinking about the population-based or public health impact of
programmes is new for many healthcare professionals. With the increasing
emphasis on cost containment and accountability, evaluation criteria such as
those in the RE-AIM model become paramount.[37] Most of our professional
training has upheld the traditional double-blind randomized clinical trial as the

'gold standard' method for evaluating interventions. While such trials have certainly advanced our knowledge, they often oversimplify clinical realities and emphasize internal validity (efficacy)[33] *at the expense of* external validity. Tunis et al.,[38] in an important paper that discusses the types of 'practical clinical trial' necessary to advance translation of research to practice, call for design and measurement issues that address concerns of clinicians and policy-makers. Especially needed is more research conducted on representative patient samples in representative clinical settings, conducted under 'real-world' conditions to help guide important policy and resource allocation decisions.[29,39]

Diabetes-specific office-based interventions

Relatively few studies of behavioural programs have been conducted in the medical office/care setting. More often, behavioural, health, lifestyle and mental health counselling have been conducted on a referral basis. Table 6.2 below and this section summarize reports of behaviour change intervention initiated or delivered in the office setting with diabetes patients, and uses the RE-AIM model to evaluate results.

Table 6.2 Summary of diabetes medical office research literature by RE-AIM issues

RE-AIM dimension	Conclusions re: state of science	Amount of research	Example diabetes references	Other chronic illness examples
Reach	Fairly broad – better than traditional education or referral	Moderate	Glasgow et al.[14,123,124]	Eakin et al.[125] Green et al.[126]
Efficacy	Variable–moderate; better for tailored interventions	Substantial	Glasgow et al.[47] McNabb[127] Greenfield et al.[44]	Strecher et al.[128] Brug et al.[129] Lorig et al.[67]
Adoption	Unknown	Little/none	Glasgow et al.[8] Glasgow et al.[84]	Goodman and Steckler[130]
Implementation	Unknown	Little	Litzelman et al.[52] Glasgow et al.[8]	Santacroce et al.[131]
Maintenance	Poor – especially unless follow-up support provided	Moderate at individual; little at clinic level	Weinberger et al.[53] Piette[31]	Wasson et al.[55]

One of the earlier psychological intervention studies to take place during regular office visits was conducted by Barbara Anderson et al.,[40] with type 1 adolescents and their family members. Adolescents randomized to the intervention attended five group visits with peers, once every 3–4 months, conducted as part of their usual medical visits, while their parents participated in concurrent group sessions with other parents. Content of the meetings focused on problem-solving and using blood glucose self-monitoring (BGSM) data for self-regulation. After 18 months, participants in the intervention condition showed significantly greater reductions in HbA1c (adjusted differences of about one per cent) than those in usual care, and more intervention adolescents than usual care adolescents (60 versus 33 per cent) reported using BGSM information when they exercised. More research is needed on similar approaches to aiding adolescents, as well as on group approaches to clinic visits for adults as have been used with success in other areas.[41,42]

A more recent intervention by this same group[43] explored the effects of a 'Care Ambassador' intervention. They randomized type 1 youth and their families to either usual care or to the Care Ambassador intervention, which focused on scheduling, confirming and documenting medical follow-up for 24 months and helping patients to negotiate the health care system. The Care Ambassador intervention significantly reduced A1c levels and lowered the hospitalization/ER use rate by half compared to the standard care. Similar, low intensity interventions have strong potential to prove cost effective, especially among high risk populations.

An example of research using a patient-activation paradigm was reported by Greenfield et al.[44] In this randomized trial, a research assistant met with patients for 20 minutes just prior to two quarterly office visits to review their medical records, discuss medical decisions and self-management issues likely to arise during that visit and rehearse negotiation and information-seeking skills. At 12-week follow-up, this patient activation intervention produced significant improvements in glucose control (adjusted differences of approximately two per cent HbA1c), days lost from work and quality of life relative to controls. Patients in the experimental condition were also significantly more active during their visit with their physician, asked more questions and elicited more information from their doctor. A recent replication of this brief counselling approach based on self-determination theory by Williams et al.[45] failed to replicate this intervention effect. In this well controlled study, a very similar patient-activation intervention was conducted in a multi-speciality diabetes care setting. The intervention was significantly more effective than the 'passive education' control condition, which consisted of watching ADA videotapes, at producing higher levels of patient involvement in objectively scored discussions with their clinicians. However, the intervention did not result in significantly better improvements in A1c levels. The authors speculated that this failure to replicate the patient activation intervention effect may have been due to the level of improvement shown by control patients (average decrease in A1c of 1.7 per cent over 12 months) in this setting, which provided intensive diabetes management.

A high tech approach to patient-centred self-management by our research group[46,47] focussed on enhancing dietary self-management. This study began by contacting all adult diabetes patients who had an upcoming visit with one of two internists. Sixty-one per cent of eligible patients agreed to participate in the study (reach), and importantly there were no differences between participants and non-participants on demographic or medical characteristics collected.[14] The intervention package involved a sequence of a 15 minute touchscreen computer assessment, which helped subjects identify dietary goals and barriers to accomplishing this goal; immediate scoring and printing of two tailored feedback/goal print-outs summarizing the information – one for the patient and one for the physician; a 20 second motivational message from the physician emphasizing the importance of the goal the patient had selected; a 15–20 minute meeting with a health educator to review the patient's goal and collaboratively develop barrier-based intervention strategies and finally two brief follow-up phone calls from the health educator to check on progress. This sequence was repeated at a 3 month follow-up visit.

Compared with a stringent, randomized control condition that received the same touchscreen computer assessment (but no tailored feedback), and physician encouragement, the intervention produced significantly greater improvements on a variety of dietary behaviour measures as well as serum cholesterol levels. More importantly, these results were maintained at essentially the same level (e.g. adjusted difference of 16 mg/dl in serum cholesterol) at a 12 month follow-up, and the intervention was found to be cost effective: an average, annual incremental cost over usual care of $115–$139 per patient and $8.40 per unit reduction in serum cholesterol level.[47]

More recently, there have been encouraging demonstrations of both low tech, office-based outreach and high tech follow-up support self-management interventions to enhance and extend usual care. Riley et al.[48] conducted a controlled pilot study in a largely Latino community health centre serving low income and uninsured patients. They evaluated and found support for an intervention designed to enhance personally tailored community support resources (based on the results of the Chronic Illness Resources Survey).[49] This intervention was found to significantly increase both use of community resources and physical activity levels among a challenged group of English and Spanish speaking patients, many but not all of whom had diabetes (they had on average 3.8 different chronic illnesses).

A more high tech approach to extending usual office based care has been evaluated in a series of studies by Piette et al.[50,51] and uses interactive voice response (IVR) technology – or automated computerized phone calls. Such systems proactively call patients at prearranged times and provide both motivational messages and self-management tips of the patient's choice, and also collect data from patients on things such as blood glucose monitoring results. A key aspect of these systems seems to be that patients understand that this is part of their care, and that the results are transmitted to clinical staff. Piette et al. have reported very encouraging controlled data that patients, and especially low income and Spanish speaking patients, will continue to use such a service over time, and that such IVR interventions significantly improve outcomes.[50,51]

Litzelman et al.[52] have provided a good example of a very low cost, office-based *system intervention*, which focused on prompting both patients and providers regarding foot care practices. Their patient intervention involved nurse–clinician meetings with one to four patients to cover foot care education, individualized behavioural contracts, telephone follow-ups at two weeks and mailed postcard reminders at 1 and 3 months. The office system intervention consisted of colurful patient folders with foot decals to identify intervention patients, prompts to ask patients to remove their footwear and a guideline-based flowsheet for physicians. One year after initiating the intervention, Litzelman et al.[52] found that this intervention package produced significant reductions in foot lesions (odds ratio = 0.4), increases in appropriate foot self-management behaviours and increases in office foot examinations (68 versus 28 per cent) compared with randomized controls. The helpfulness of follow-up support was also demonstrated by Weinberger et al.[53] who found that brief telephone calls conducted by nurses led to reductions in glycosylated haemoglobin. In a randomized study with older type 2 VA patients, they found that calls conducted an average of once a month significantly decreased Ghb levels (adjusted difference of 0.6 per cent) relative to usual care. These results are consistent with studies demonstrating the efficacy and cost-effectiveness of telephone calls for enhancing maintenance and even serving as alternatives to office visits for non-diabetes, health-related issues.[54,55]

Finally, both the Diabetes Control and Complications Trial (DCCT)[56] and the Diabetes Prevention Program (DPP)[32] provide interesting examples of the power of systematically reorganizing office practices and patient self-management support activities. Although often interpreted solely as demonstrations of the efficacy of intensive management, the DCCT and DPP obtained their incredibly good adherence (implementation) and low attrition rates by providing an impressive array of ongoing patient support activities.[1,57] These trials are interesting because they are also the best example of well conducted and extremely influential efficacy trials in diabetes. They unquestionably produced impressive clinical outcomes. However, review of the controversies and differences of opinion regarding the applicability of DCCT- and DPP-like procedures[58,59] illustrates the difficulties of making practice guideline and resource allocation decisions based solely on efficacy trials. From the RE-AIM perspective, these trials maximized efficacy and implementation results, but would receive low scores on reach (percentage and representativeness of patients participating) and adoption (conducted predominantly in unrepresentative, specialized tertiary care centres and with very high levels of clinical expertise and resources). More effectiveness trials conducted in primary care settings using more representative, practical population-based approaches and outcomes are needed.[11,29,34,38]

An example of such a study was recently reported by Glasgow and colleagues,[8] who recruited 52 primary care physicians and their regular office staff members to participate in a randomized quality improvement project. The intervention was initiated in the waiting room when patients came for primary care visits related to diabetes. The study involved 886 type 2 diabetes patients (75 per cent of those contacted and invited to participate from lists of all type 2 patients in these offices took part). Intervention patients completed a touchscreen computer program that assisted them and the staff to set priorities for care and to establish behaviour change goals for dietary, physical activity or smoking change. The computer program provided a separate tailored print-out for the patient, the physician and the office care manager (usually a nurse). The control condition involved completing many of the same measures on a touchscreen computer, but the print-out focused on general health risk information – such as risky drinking, wearing seat belts and getting cancer screenings – not directly related to diabetes self-management.

The programme was well implemented and 90–100 per cent of patients received the computer intervention, met with the office manager, went over the print-out with their physician and received at least one follow-up phone call. Relative to the control condition, the intervention significantly improved the percentage of both recommended laboratory assays and patient-centred behavioural counselling that patients received. Also, the intervention was equally effective across a variety of patient subgroups, including Latinos, older patients, those with less education and those with no previous computer experience. This practical trial demonstrated that regular office staff can consistently deliver a computer-assisted intervention and improve the quality of care that patients receive. Other outcomes important for practical clinical trials[29,38] including biological outcomes, behaviour change and quality of life will be collected at later follow-up assessments.

Examples from other areas

Although the evidence from medical office-based interventions with diabetes patients is promising, it is still preliminary. Therefore, it is useful to consider interventions that have been successful in utilizing or supplementing the medical office encounter to enhance patient outcomes in other chronic illnesses. Below, I review several such examples that should transfer to diabetes.

The work of the Stanford Cardiac Rehabilitation Program[60] with patients who have suffered a recent heart attack serves as a model of how integrated, office- and home-based self-management support can be provided. Their programme is based on the social cognitive theory[61] components of individualized goal setting, feedback and follow-up support integrated with medical care and coordinated by a nurse case manager.

This study evaluated computer-assisted goal setting, self-management planning and follow-up telephone calls conceptually similar to the programme employed in diabetes by Glasgow et al.[47,62] This multiple risk factor reduction programme was found to be significantly better in facilitating smoking cessation (70 versus 53 per cent, $p = 0.03$), physical fitness increases (9.3 versus 8.4 METS, $p = .001$) and lowering lipid levels (LDL cholesterol 107 versus 132 mg/dl, $p = .001$) than a usual care condition in a randomized trial with 585 recent heart disease patients.

An innovative approach to redesigning the medical office visit has been employed with older chronic illness patients[42] in the Kaiser Permanente Colorado system. Rather than seeing patients in the usual 10–15 minute individual session, primary care is provided via monthly 90 minute group visits. These sessions, co-led by the physician and nurse coordinator, incorporate vital sign assessments, medication checks and other elements of care into the group session which also permits discussion of various self-management topics of interest to the group, and much opportunity for peer support. Beck *et al.*[42] evaluated this approach relative to traditional physician–patient dyadic care in a 1 year randomized trial with 321 seniors having chronic illnesses. They found that the group visit participants had fewer ER visits, visits to sub-specialists and repeat hospitalizations. Both patients and physicians reported greater satisfaction with the group visits, which cost an overall average of $15 per month less per member. Wagner *et al.*[63] and Sadur *et al.*[64] have recently demonstrated the generality of this approach and its applicability for diabetes by replicating success with this group visit model of providing primary care for diabetes patients.

Approaches to *extending* the self-management support provided in the office have been developed by Lorig *et al.*[65] and Leveille *et al.*[66] Lorig and colleagues have developed a peer-led arthritis, self-management programme and found it to be superior to usual care in a series of randomized trials. Recently, they have reported 4 year follow-up results demonstrating lasting reductions in pain, physician visits and cost relative to comparison conditions, and adapted their programme, which emphasizes self-efficacy enhancement,[61] for diabetes patients and for patients having a variety of chronic illnesses, with similar impressive results on health care utilization.[67]

Leveille *et al.*[66] demonstrated the value of community support to complement primary care in a randomized trial of 201 chronically ill, frail adults age 70 and older. Their disability prevention, disease self-management intervention conducted in a senior centre in collaboration with primary care providers produced less decline in function on standardized instruments and fewer disability days than controls. In addition, the intervention condition participants became more physically active, significantly reduced their psychoactive medication use, and had fewer in-patient hospital days.

Computer technology has been used to supplement office care and provides examples of cost-effective strategies for providing tailored goal setting, skills training and support. Skinner *et al.*[68] had primary care patients complete telephone interviews. Female patients age 40–65 who had visited their primary care provider within the past 2 years were randomized to receive a posted tailored health communication based on their mammography history, beliefs, risk status and perceived barriers, or to a standardized letter encouraging mammography. This brief, single contact intervention improved mammography rates among women who were due for screening compared with standardized letters (44 versus 31 per cent overall). Significant interaction effects revealed that the intervention was especially effective with African American women and with lower income women.[68] A similar approach to enhancing adherence to diabetes care guidelines might be tested.

Gustafson *et al.*[69] presented the first randomized outcome evaluation of an Internet health information/support system for patients. Their CHESS (Comprehensive Health Enhancement Support System) interactive computer support system, which has also been applied with breast cancer, heart disease and problem-drinking patients, was evaluated for its ability to provide support for HIV-positive patients. Half of the 204 patients had computers linked to the CHESS system placed in their homes for 3 or 6 months; controls received no intervention beyond usual care. The CHESS system was used daily, and produced significant improvements in several quality-of-life dimensions and fewer and shorter hospitalizations than were seen in control patients. The Internet, in particular, as well as other interactive health technologies, have considerable potential – if appropriately developed and implemented – to enhance, inform and streamline patient–provider interactions.[4,31] These technologies are by no means 'magic bullets', but they may be especially effective in helping patients become more informed about their care, and in providing support and motivation between office visits.

Many of the self-management interventions above have been validated in large-scale randomized studies with patient populations traditionally considered to be challenging (heart disease, older adults with multiple illnesses, arthritis, HIV/ AIDS patients). Common elements across these diverse interventions seem to be a patient-centred approach that individualizes self-management and goal setting, provides strategies and models for coping with barriers and importantly some form of follow-up support that either changes or supplements that available through usual primary care. These strategies are the key components of 'the cycle of self-management' (see Figure 6.2), and should also be successful, with appropriate adaptation, in diabetes.

Training other clinicians in self-management

Bob Anderson, Martha Funnell and colleagues[70] have reported on the results of a training programme for diabetes educators to help them learn patient empowerment strategies (see Chapter 5). They evaluated a three-day skills based workshop (these authors have subsequently also developed shorter training programmes), which included following a simulated diabetes care regimen prior to the workshop training, demonstrations and practice in empowerment counselling skills and finally a videotape review of counselling sessions. Following training, participants in the workshop showed significant improvement from baseline in counselling skills (on both videotape simulations and audio recordings of actual counselling sessions), and in their attitudes toward supporting patient autonomy on the Diabetes Attitudes Scale.[70] An interesting outcome of the study was that several

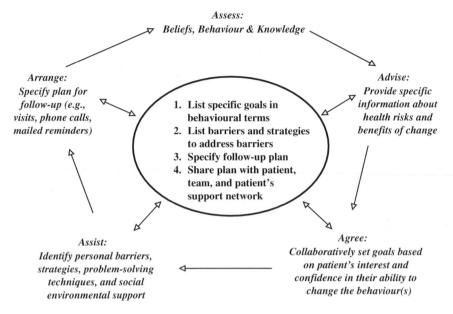

Figure 6.2   '5 As' model of self-management

of the educators who participated in the programme have, in turn, presented counselling skill in-service programmes to colleagues. The empowerment approach has been demonstrated to produce better patient outcomes than usual care in a randomized trial.[71] More research on the empowerment model and related approaches such as motivational interviewing[72] are needed, especially studies that evaluate the adoption (who participates in such training), implementation and maintenance of counselling skills.

A number of diabetes quality improvement 'collaboratives' have been conducted since 1999 that have included a prominent role for self-management. These collaboratives consist of a series of learning sessions typically conducted over a period of 12 months, interspersed with action periods during which participating health care teams test out new care innovations. The majority of the collaboratives that feature self-management are based on the evidence-based Chronic Care Model of Wagner and colleagues,[73–76] which emphasizes that chronic illness care needs to be patient-centred, proactive, planned and population based. Preliminary reports from collaboratives sponsored by the Robert Wood Johnson Foundation and the Bureau of Primary Health Care, which includes community and migrant health centres in the US that serve uninsured and low income patients, have been encouraging.[77,78] Controlled studies are needed (and more comprehensive evaluation is being conducted by the RAND corporation; see www.rand.org/health/ICICE), but it appears that teams from a wide range of health care systems can produce care improvements across the panel of patients they see (not just those who are highly motivated to volunteer for education or a research study).

Most evaluations[79,80] have found substantial improvement in the rate at which collaboratively set self-management goals are recorded in patient medical records. The '5 As' model of self-management described above has been widely used to train teams in self-management. It appears that community health centres and other low resourced settings can successfully implement these changes and that the teams that are most successful at self-management distribute support activities across a variety of team members (rather than relying primarily on the physician to do everything) and conduct a number of 'rapid cycle experiments' or tests of innovative activities, rather than trying to plan a perfect improvement programme prior to implementation. Recent articles by Glasgow and colleagues share self-management lessons learned from these collaborative approaches to staff and medical office behaviour change.[79,81]

6.4   Target Groups for Inclusion/Exclusion

From the existing literature, it is not possible to draw firm conclusions about subgroups for whom office-based interventions are most effective. More research is needed on patient characteristics, on characteristics of the patient's social and physical environment[1,82,83] and on medical office and staff characteristics associated with success.

There are likely some subsets of patients who have very complex or challenging issues that require more intensive intervention than is usually possible in the typical office visit. Such groups would include newly diagnosed patients, those with major psychological disorders and those being started on intensive insulin management regimens. Referral to appropriate specialists or more intensive programmes is warranted in such cases. When using referrals or centralized disease management services located outside the primary care office, it is especially important to have good two-way communication and to ensure that the patient is given consistent messages about goals and strategies.

It is encouraging that the studies conducted to date have generally found office-based behavioural strategies to be equally effective across gender, age, education and medical/diabetes history and severity levels.[84,85] Also, contrary to stereotypes about the 'digital divide', available data seem to indicate that patients without computer experience do as well as other patients.[8,84,85] However, more medical office-related research is needed with adolescents, with socioeconomically disadvantaged patients, and on group visit formats[42,63,64] for delivering primary care (as contrasted with separate referrals to outside diabetes education groups, which are not well attended and have numerous barriers to participation).

Areas in need of future research are the relationship of health literacy[86] and numeracy to outcomes, and the effect of potential patient and office practice

moderating variables on outcomes such as reach, implementation and maintenance. In general, it appears that office-based behavioural assessment and
counselling strategies can be effective for the vast majority of diabetes patients.
Office-based psychosocial interventions can be used as the first stage in a stepped
care programme[87] and have few, if any, contraindications.

6.5 Assessment and Clinic Flow

As depicted in Figures 6.1 and 6.3, there are many factors that influence diabetes
self-management and its outcomes. The left-hand side of Figure 6.3 illustrates the
multiple levels of factors that influence diabetes self-management. The centre of

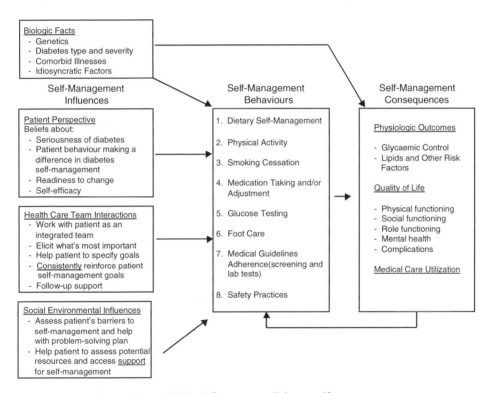

Figure 6.3 Multiple influences on diabetes self-management

the figure contains the various components of diabetes self-management. These
component tasks are listed separately to illustrate that there is usually little
relationship between the extent to which a patient follows one aspect of the
regimen and their level of self-management in other areas. Finally, the right-hand
side of the figure depicts the consequences of self-management, including
physiologic, quality of life and health care utilization outcomes. It is important

to stress that self-management and diabetes control are not the same; self-management is one of the multiple determinants of health outcomes (along with genetics, regimen and medication prescriptions, stress, comorbidities, disease severity and other variables).[88–90] One cannot judge a patient's level of self-management from their HbA1c level. Poor metabolic control indicates that something is wrong, but it does not give specific information about what is wrong.[16] Also, good diabetes outcomes and adjustment involve more than just low HbA1c levels: variables such as the patient's cardiovascular risk factors (smoking status, blood pressure, lipids), mental health status and social, physical and role functioning (i.e. health-related quality of life) are equally or more important outcomes.[91–95]

Patient factors

The most important factors in developing self-management goals are the patient's perspective on the diabetes regimen and what changes she or he considers reasonable and realistic. Two important beliefs are that patients (1) consider their diabetes to be serious and (2) believe that what they do will make a difference.[96–98] Patients who do not hold these beliefs will likely not be motivated to engage in self-management behaviours. Such patients may need additional personalized feedback on the specific implications of diabetes for their health as well as education on the potential benefits of specific self-management behaviours. The books *The Human Side of Diabetes* by Michael Raymond[18] and *Psyching Out Diabetes* by Rubin *et al.*[99] are useful resources for both patients and clinicians in illustrating how common experiences in living with diabetes can either promote or interfere with establishment of such beliefs. In particular, it is important to see whether a patient considers lifestyle aspects of diabetes management (e.g. diet and exercise; not smoking) as important as medical aspects (e.g. medication taking and glucose testing). If the patient does not, he or she will be unlikely to follow through with the challenges of lifestyle modification.

Health care team issues

Consistency and reinforcement of patient goals across different health care team members is paramount. Rather than having the physician emphasize medication, the nurse stress glucose testing and the nutritionist recommend major dietary changes, all team members need to reinforce a common self-management behaviour for that visit. The Litzelman *et al.*[52] study provides a good example of how to coordinate preventive foot care activities, including brief education while patients are waiting to see the physician, having the nurse ask the patient to remove their shoes and socks before the physician arrives, followed by a physician foot examination and reinforcement of the patient education message about foot care. The patient needs to leave a given visit with a clear idea and a written 'goal' or 'action plan' of the key goal(s) for the next visit, and an understanding of why the goal is important to the management of their diabetes (see the example in Figure 6.4). When patients are given assignments, it is particularly important to review and comment at the next contact on their progress and any records that the patient has kept. The 1994 issue of *Diabetes Spectrum* edited by Anderson and Jenkins[100] on educational innovations provides discussion of other issues in system-wide interventions, as does the special supplement to *Diabetes Care* edited by Mazze and Etzwiler[101] and the conceptual article by Jenkins.[91]

Overcoming Barriers to Self-Management

For: **Mr. Jones**　　　　　　　　　　　　Date: **12/12/04**

Personalized Goal for Next Few Months:

To:　**Substitute low-fat foods for high-fat foods (for example, use nonfat mayonnaise instead of regular mayonnaise.)**

Specific Plans for Accomplishing this Goal:

1. _____ –
2. _____ –
3. _____ –

Type of Situation That Is Most Challenging:
Moods and feelings that lead to eating

Specific Situations:
I feel down or blue.
I am bored or restless and feel like snacking.

Other Situations Which Make It Difficult:

I have difficulty finding low-fat food items where I shop.

I have junk food around the house.

How You Can Prepare for Problem Situations

1. _____
2. _____
3. _____

---

*NOTE: In this example, information in bold was printed by computerized assessment, Blanks are to be filled in by patient and educator.

Figure 6.4　Example self-management action plan

The social environment

It is important to assess and incorporate both the patients' anticipated barriers to self-management and their available resources, at the level of (1) family and friends and (2) broader community influences including work and neighbourhood factors (see Figures 6.1 and 6.3).[102] This can be accomplished by asking the patient what s/he thinks might interfere with the identified self-management goal(s) (e.g., 'Ms. Smith, what things do you think might make it difficult for you to follow the eating plan we developed?'). The clinician can then help the patient develop possible solutions, focusing on the use of available family, friend or community resources. Most communities have available a series of free or low cost support or reinforcement activities (e.g. senior centre or YMCA activity programmes, ADA meetings, hospital or HMO education programmes) that can extend the motivation patients receive during office visits. Anderson and Funnell[17] have provided a useful discussion and examples of community support options to reinforce physician messages about diabetes management, and Anderson *et al.*[103] have described a series of publicly available camera ready, two-page, single-issue newsletters that can be sent to patients to reinforce a selected goal.

Self-management activities do not occur in a vacuum, but rather in a social context. If maintenance of self-management is to be expected, follow-up support must be arranged in the form of family and community social support,[48] and follow-up contacts with members of the health care team.[55] The flow chart (Figure 6.5) and text below address how these suggestions might work into the flow of a busy practice.

Prior to the visit

Materials, surveys, or reminders posted to the patient prior to the visit can help focus attention on the importance of patient behaviour and inform the visit. One such example is a reminder to the patient to bring information monitored between visits (e.g. blood glucose, food intake or exercise logs), and to have them update their status on recommended guidelines[104] or other 'best practices'.

The waiting room

The focus on self-management should continue while the patient is in the waiting room. The patient's attention can be drawn to the importance of self-management activities by having various pamphlets, posters and notices placed in the waiting room. These might include notices from the hospital or clinic regarding diabetes education or information classes and support groups, as well as tailored

> ### Prior to Visit
>
> Mailed reminder re: goal set last visit,
> self-monitoring records
> (e.g., blood glucose, diet, exercise),
> recommended lab tests.

> ### Waiting Room
>
> Patient completes Self-Management Form
> or computer assessment.
>
> Surrounded by information on diabetes self-management
> (pamphlets, posters, notices).

> ### Exam Room and Vital Signs
>
> Nurse gives patient feedback on changes since last visit
> (blood glucose, weight, blood pressure, lipids).
>
> Inquires about self-management goal since last visit.
>
> Nurse checks Self-Management Form and asks which area is currently of most concern
> (circles area for physician; reinforces patient interest;
> educates on importance of self-care).

> ### Physician Exam
>
> Check Self-Management Form and discuss area of most concern to patient.
>
> Message: "I see you would most like to discuss…Diabetes is serious
> and your behaviour is important in managing it."
>
> Reinforce patient's willingness to change behaviour and
> refer to nurse or CDE for specific plan.

> ### Nurse or CDE Follow-up
>
> Review and clarify goals for behaviour change in one area of self-care.
>
> Develop specific, realistic, measurable plan.
>
> Have patient identify barriers to goal and assist in problem-solving.
>
> Plan for continued support: refer to diabetes education or support group;
> community resources; phone call between visits, etc.
>
> Record goal (with copy for patient) and plan for follow-up at subsequent contacts.

Figure 6.5 Flow of brief office-based diabetes self-management intervention

pamphlets, CD-ROMs or videos on weight management, exercise or smoking cessation.

While patients are waiting, they can complete a brief form assessing their current level of diabetes self-management activities. An example of such a form is given in Figure 6.6. This assessment could be easily conducted using a computer

1. Which of the following has your health care team (doctor, nurse, dietician, or diabetes educator) advised you to do? Please check all that apply:
    __a. Follow a low-fat eating plan.
    __b. Reduce the number of calories you eat.
    __c. Eat 5 or more servings per day of fruits and vegetables.
    __d. Eat very few sweets.
    __e. Other (specify): _____
    __f. I have not been given any advice about my diet.

2. How often did you follow your recommended eating plan since your last visit?
    ___Always ___Usually ___Sometimes ___Rarely ___Never

3. Which of the following has your health care team (doctor, nurse, dietician, or diabetes educator) advised you to do? Please check all that apply:
    __a. Do low to moderate activity (such as walking) on a daily basis.
    __b. Exercise continuously for at least 20 minutes at least 3 times a week.
    __c. Fit physical activity into your daily routine (take stairs instead of elevators, park a block away and walk, etc.).
    __d. Other (specify): _____
    __e. I have not been given advice about physical activity.

4. How often did you follow your exercise plan recommendations since your last visit?
    ___Always ___Usually ___Sometimes ___Rarely ___Never

5. Which of the following has your health care team (doctor, nurse, dietician, or diabetes educator) advised you to do? Please check all that apply:
    __a. Test your blood glucose (sugar) using a drop of blood from your finger.
    __b. Test your blood glucose using a machine to read the results.
    __c. Test your urine for sugar.
    __d. Other (specify): _____
    __e. I have not been given advice about testing my blood glucose.

6. How often are you supposed to test your blood glucose level?
    __ times per day or __ times per week

7. How often did you follow your blood glucose testing recommendations since your last visit?
    ___Always ___Usually ___Sometimes ___Rarely ___Never

8. Which of the following medications for your diabetes has your doctor prescribed? Please check all that apply:
    __a. An insulin shot 1 or 2 times a day.
    __b. An insulin shot 3 or more times a day.
    __c. Diabetes pills (sulfa drugs) to control your blood glucose level.
    __d. Glucophage (Metformin tablets)
    __e. Other (specify): _____
    __f. I have not been prescribed medication for my diabetes.

9. How often did you take your diabetes medication as prescribed since your last visit?
    ___Always ___Usually ___Sometimes ___Rarely ___Never

10. Which of the following has your health care team (doctor, nurse, dietician, or diabetes educator) advised you to do? Please check all that apply:
    __a. Check your feet daily for sores, cuts, calluses, infection, etc.
    __b. Check inside your shoes daily for loose objects or rough edges.
    __c. Not to go barefoot either inside or outdoors.
    __d. Wash your feet daily, remembering to dry between your toes.
    __e. Other (specify): _____
    __f. I have not been given advice about foot care.

11.   How often did you follow your foot care recommendations since your last visit?
      ___Always ___Usually ___Sometimes ___Rarely ___Never

12.   Have you smoked, even a puff, during the past 7 days?
      ___Yes   ___No (skip to Question #15)

13.   Has anyone from your health care team advised you to stop smoking?
      ___Yes   ___No

14.   Are you seriously considering stopping smoking in the near future?
      ___Yes   ___No

15.   Has your health care team instructed you what to do if your blood glucose is too low or too high?
                  ___Yes   ___No

16.   How confident are you that you know what to do if your blood glucose is too low?
          Not confident   Confident
              1   2   3   4   5   6   7
17.   How confident are you that you know what to do if your blood glucose is too high?
          Not confident   Confident
              1   2   3   4   5   6   7

      (NOTE: We recommend assessment of barriers to achieving goals in the area(s) in which patients are having difficulty)

      © Oregon Research Institute and Group Health Cooperative, 1995

Figure 6.6   Diabetes self-management and patient involvement assessment form

set up in a corner of the waiting room. The assessment information could also be incorporated into an interactive health technology intervention.[8,47] Information from the self-management form is then used during the remainder of the visit, as described below.

The examination room and vital signs

When the nurse or other office staff member takes the patient to the examination room and assesses vital signs (which should include smoking status),[105,106] this provides an opportunity to give the patient feedback on key issues such as weight gain or loss and changes in blood glucose, cholesterol or blood pressure since the last visit. The nurse can also briefly check the self-management form and any other monitoring records for completeness and ask the patient which self-management area he or she would most like to focus on during this visit (circling the area for the physician and reinforcing the patient for willingness to work on diabetes self-management, or educating the patient about the importance of self-management). This is also an excellent opportunity to identify often neglected issues, such as depression, stress, smoking or foot care.

Physician examination

The physician should begin by asking the patient what they would most like to discuss at that visit.[17,46] The two most important messages from the physician have to do with the seriousness of diabetes and the importance of patient behaviour in managing the disease. Following up on the self-management form, the physician should address the area of greatest concern to the patient. This is an opportunity both to reinforce the patient's intention to make behaviour changes and to educate the patient on the centrality of self-management (e.g. 'Mrs. Gonzales, I'm glad to see that you'd like to focus on your eating. Following a low saturated fat diet will help you to better manage your diabetes and will also reduce your risk of heart disease'). The physician can then let the patient know that the nurse, dietitian, diabetes educator or psychologist will meet with them briefly after the examination to help them develop a specific plan for making changes in the self-management area.

Follow-up

Following the examination, the nurse or diabetes educator meets briefly with the patient to review and clarify specific goals for behaviour change and develop problem-solving strategies. It is critical – and often inadequately implemented – to consider the patient's perspective and readiness to change during this process. Anderson and colleagues have written extensively on patient empowerment and patient-centred approaches to enhancing diabetes self-management.[17,70] Patients will be unlikely to make behaviour changes if (1) they are not motivated to do so, (2) they do not understand the importance of the recommended behaviour in managing their diabetes or (3) they do not have the necessary skills to carry out the behaviour. Optimally, the goal(s) should be generated by the patient and then worked into a specific behavioural plan in collaboration with the educator (or interactive technology aid). Using principles of behaviour change, this means that the goal(s) should be specific, manageable and measurable, that the patient should understand the importance of the behaviour in managing diabetes and that he or she should be educated in the skills necessary to perform the behaviour.[107–112]

Once a plan for a specific behaviour change is agreed upon, the next step is to ask the patient to identify the things that are most likely to interfere with following the plan. Help the patient to come up with at least two practical solutions to these barriers. One of the most common barriers to self-management, even for very motivated patients, is functioning in a home, work, and neighbourhood environment that does not support the self-management goal. (There are brief questionnaires that can be used to structure this discussion).[113,114,116] A number of studies have evaluated patients' 'barriers' to self-management.[113,115,116] Rather than labelling the patient as non-compliant, an attempt should be made to understand the factors that interfere with the identified goal. Commonly reported barriers include lack of family support, stress, being busy, being away from home, lack of insurance reimbursement (e.g. for glucose testing strips) and lack of convenient, safe, low-cost places to exercise. Most patients experience the highest frequency of barriers to dietary and exercise adherence and the fewest to medication taking.[114,115,117]

Finally, it is also important to assist the patient in accessing support for their new behaviour.[48] This might entail referral to diabetes education classes or a support group, related reading materials and often a follow-up or IVR phone call to check on progress between visits.[31,51,53] Finally, the self-management goal and plan for achieving it should be recorded (Figure 6.4), with a copy given to the patient and another placed in the chart so that it can be referred to at the next contact.

6.6   Links to Medical Management

A key advantage of office-based psychosocial interventions is potential for coordination with and integration into regular clinical practice. Behavioural and psychosocial issues can be addressed by health care staff and seen by patients as a regular part of patient care. This is in contrast to the situation in most settings, in which a 'psychological or self-management' referral is seen as stigmatizing, separate from usual patient care and often poorly connected with the medical management of diabetes.

Just because an intervention is conducted in the office setting is no guarantee that it will be integrated with other aspects of a patient's care. It is essential that all health care team members be aware of what other team members are working on with a patient, that they reinforce each other's efforts and that they do not overwhelm the patient with too many goals and priorities at once. Such coordination and mutual support is much more likely to happen if it is programmed into the office practice[8,118] and prompted by the use of patient goal setting and action plan forms (Figure 6.4).

As reviewed above, there are different models for determining which staff member implements the various behavioural strategies, and these actions need to be tailored to the particular office setting.[81,118] To maximize consistent and quality implementation, most intensive behavioural interventions should be delivered either by behavioural specialists experienced in diabetes and working in health care settings, by diabetes educators trained in behavioural intervention or by user friendly, interactive computer-based applications.

It is also clear that one does not need to be a highly trained psychologist to deliver most of the behavioural intervention strategies recommended above. The few studies that have evaluated counsellor characteristics have not found one type of health professional to be more effective than others at producing behaviour change.[85] This assumes that staff members are well trained, and receive adequate supervision and feedback. From a social influence perspective, it makes most sense to have a physician deliver the intervention. In practice, this is seldom possible due to the extreme time limitations[19] and lack of behavioural training of physicians.[117] In most cases, the doctor probably best serves as a motivator who can briefly emphasize the importance of behavioural goals and of working with the behavioral interventionist. The most generalizable model is probably to have some form of automated or rapidly scored assessment, followed by a motivational message from the physician, and then intervention and follow-up conducted by a nurse or case manager.

The greatest opportunity for linking to medical management and improving overall quality of diabetes care lies in the area of tracking performance indices for preventive care[119] for all patients in an office practice. This requires an accurate diabetes registry and a list of best practices that includes behavioural, psychosocial and patient-focussed issues[7] in addition to medical and laboratory screening activities. The second most important issue, and one that has impressive empirical support, is to conduct brief follow-up contacts with patients as discussed above.

6.7   Unanswered Questions, New Directions

Good progress has been made in medical office-based psychosocial interventions during the few years that this has been investigated, but much remains to be learned. As summarized in Tables 6.1 and 6.2, studies are particularly needed of the extent and characteristics of practices that adopt, implement and maintain such interventions. This conclusion is not unique to medical office-based interventions, but also applies to much of health promotion.[34,36] As research shifts to a broader focus that includes not only individual and intrapersonal determinants of health and behaviour, but also broader social–environmental determinants, setting and organization factors become an important area of investigation.[118,120] As this field of inquiry advances, the issues studied will shift from basic questions, such as 'does this type of intervention work?' to more sophisticated questions, such as 'What type of intervention is most effective for what purpose (e.g. increasing participation; producing immediate behaviour change; enhancing maintenance) with which type of patient in which type of setting when implemented by what type of interventionist?'. Given the inherent advantages of consistent delivery, freeing staff time for other duties, automated and immediate scoring and feedback and the high degree of individualization possible, we are likely to see much more application of interactive computer-based applications in medical settings.[4] It is hoped that these applications will be evidence based, and that they will be developed with a focus on the RE-AIM dimensions discussed above to broaden their public health impact.

The final and most important challenge for the future remains optimal ways in which to integrate psychosocial assessments and interventions into regular medical office-based diabetes care, and to do so in a way that enhances efficiency, quality of care and patient-centred outcomes.[121,122]

References

1. Glasgow RE, Fisher EB, Anderson BJ *et al*. Behavioral science in diabetes: contributions and opportunities. *Diabetes Care* 1999; **22**: 832–843.
2. Glasgow RE, McKay HG, Boles SM, Vogt TM. Interactive technology, behavioral science, and family practice. *J Fam Pract* 1999; **48**: 464–470.
3. Street RL Jr, Gold WR, Manning TE. Health promotion and interactive technology: Theoretical applications and future directions. London: Erlbaum, 1997.
4. Glasgow RE, Bull SS, Piette JD, Steiner J. Interactive behavior change technology: A partial solution to the competing demands of primary care. *Am J Prev Med* 2004; **27** (25): 80–87.
5. Harris MI. Medical care for patients with diabetes: Epidemiologic aspects. *Ann Intern Med* 1996; **124**: 117–122.
6. Marrero DG. Current effectiveness of diabetes health care in the U.S. *Diabetes Rev* 1994; **2**: 292–309.
7. Glasgow RE, Boles SM, Calder D, Dreyer L, Bagdade J. Diabetes care practices in primary care: Results from two samples and three performance indices. *Diabetes Educ* 1999; **25**: 755–763.
8. Glasgow RE, Nutting PA, King DK *et al*. Results from a practical randomized trial of the Diabetes Priority Program: Improvements in care and patient outcomes using RE-AIM criteria. *J Gen Intern Med* 2004; **19** (12): 1167–1174.
9. Glasgow RE. A practical model of diabetes management and education. *Diabetes Care* 1995; **18**: 117–126.
10. Winett RA, King AC, Altman DG. *Health Psychology and Public Health: an Integrative Approach*. New York: Pergamon, 1989.
11. Glasgow RE, Wagner E, Kaplan RM, Vinicor F, Smith L, Norman J. If diabetes is a public health problem, why not treat it as one? A population-based approach to chronic illness. *Ann Behav Med* 1999; **21**: 159–170.
12. Funnell MM, Anderson RM. Patient education in the physician's office. *Pract Diabetol* 1993; **12**: 22–25.
13. Wagner EH. Population-based management of diabetes care. *Patient Educ Couns* 1995; **26**: 225–230.
14. Glasgow RE, Eakin EG, Toobert DJ. How generalizable are the results of diabetes self-management research? The impact of participation and attrition. *Diabetes Educ* 1996; **22**: 573–585.
15. National Institutes of Health. *Diabetes in America*, NIH Publication No. 95-1468. Bethesda, MD: National Institute of Diabetes and Digestive and Kidney Diseases, 1995.
16. Johnson SB. Regimen adherence: Roles and responsibilities of health care providers. *Diabetes Spectrum* 1993; **6**: 204–205.
17. Anderson RM, Funnell MM. The role of the physician in patient education. *Pract Diabetol* 1990; **9**: 10–12.
18. Raymond M. *The Human Side of Diabetes: Beyond Doctors, Diets and Drugs*. Chicago, IL: Noble, 1992.
19. Stange KC, Woolf SH, Gjeltema K. One minute for prevention: The power of leveraging to fulfill the promise of health behavior counseling. *Am J Prev Med* 2002; **22**: 320–323.

20. Yarnell KS, Pollack KI, Ostbye T, Krause KM, Michener JL. Primary care: Is there enough time for prevention? *Am J Public Health* 2003; **93**: 635–641.

21. Orlandi MA. Promoting health and preventing disease in health care settings: An analysis of barriers. *Prev Med* 1987; **16**: 119–130.

22. Oregon Diabetes Project. *Measuring Quality of Care in Health Systems: Population-Based Guidelines for Diabetes Mellitus.* Portland, OR: State of Oregon, 1997.

23. American Diabetes Association Task Force to Revise the National Standards. National standards for diabetes self-management education programs. *Diabetes Care* 1995; **18**: 141–143.

24. American Diabetes Association. Standards of medical care for patients with diabetes mellitus. *Diabetes Care* 1997; **20**: S5–S13.

25. American Diabetes Association. *Mission Statement* 1995.

26. Harris MI, Eastman RC, Siebert C. The DCCT and medical care for diabetes in the U.S. *Diabetes Care* 1994; **17**: 761–764.

27. Anderson BJ, Rubin RRE. *Practical Psychology for Diabetes Clinicians: How to Deal With the Key Behavioral Issues Faced by Patients and Health Care Teams.* Alexandria, VA: American Diabetes Association, 2002.

28. McCulloch DK, Glasgow RE, Hampson SE, Wagner E. A systematic approach to diabetes management in the post-DCCT era. *Diabetes Care* 1994; **17**: 765–769.

29. Glasgow RE. Translating research to practice: Lessons learned, areas for improvement, and future directions. *Diabetes Care* 2003; **26**: 2451–2456.

30. Glasgow RE, Bull SS. Making a difference with interactive technology: Considerations in using and evaluating computerized aids for diabetes self-management education. *Diabetes Spectrum* 2001; **14**: 99–106.

31. Piette J. Enhancing support via interactive technologies. *Curr Diabetes Rep* 2002; **2**: 160–165.

32. Knowler WC, Barrett-Connor E, Fowler SE *et al.* Reduction in the incidence of type 2 diabetes with lifestyle intervention or metformin. *N Engl J Med* 2002; **346**: 393–403.

33. Flay BR. Efficacy and effectiveness trials (and other phases of research) in the development of health promotion programs. *Prev Med* 1986; **15**: 451–474.

34. Glasgow RE, Vogt TM, Boles SM. Evaluating the public health impact of health promotion interventions: The RE-AIM framework. *Am J Public Health* 1999; **89**: 1322–1327.

35. Glasgow RE, Bull SS, Gillette C, Klesges LM, Dzewaltowski DA. Behavior change intervention research in health care settings: A review of recent reports with emphasis on external validity. *Am J Prev Med* 2002; **23**: 62–69.

36. Glasgow RE, Klesges LM, Dzewaltowski DA, Bull SS, Estabrooks P. The future of health behavior change research: What is needed to improve translation of research into health promotion practice? *Ann Behav Med* 2004; **27**: 3–12.

37. Glasgow RE, Klesges LM, Dzewaltowski DA, Estabrooks PA, Vogt TM. Evaluating the overall impact of health promotion programs: Using the RE-AIM framework for decision making and to consider complex issues. *Health Educ Res* in press.

38. Tunis SR, Stryer DB, Clancey CM. Practical clinical trials. Increasing the value of clinical research for decision making in clinical and health policy. *JAMA* 2003; **290**: 1624–1632.

39. Glasgow RE. Trial report–Psychological aspects. Making it real: translation research on the difficult issues. *Curr Diabetes Rep* 2003; **3**: 125–126.

40. Anderson BJ, Wolf FM, Burkhart MT, Cornell RG, Bacon GE. Effects of peer-group intervention on metabolic control of adolescents with IDDM: Randomized outpatient study. *Diabetes Care* 1989; **12**: 179–183.

41. Wagner EH. Care of older people with chronic illness. In Calkins E, Boult C, Wagner EH, Pacala J (eds), *New Ways to Care for Older People.* New York: Springer, 1998, pp 39–64.

42. Beck A, Scott J, Williams P *et al.* A randomized trial of group outpatient visits for chronically ill older HMO members: The cooperative health care clinic. *JAGS* 1997; **45**: 543–549.

43. Laffell LM, Brackett J, Ho J, Anderson BJ. Changing the process of diabetes care improves metabolic outcomes and reduces hospitalizations. *Quality Management Health Care* 1998; **6**: 53–62.

44. Greenfield S, Kaplan SH, Ware JE, Yano EM, Frank H. Patients' participation in medical care: Effects on blood sugar control and quality of life in diabetes. *J Gen Intern Med* 1988; **3**: 448–457.

45. Williams GC, McGregor HA, Zeldman A, Freedman ZR, Elder D, Deci EL. Promoting glycemic control through diabetes self-management: Evaluating a patient activation intervention. *Patient Educ Couns* 2005; **56** (1): 28–34.

46. Glasgow RE, Toobert DJ, Hampson SE. Effects of a brief office-based intervention to facilitate diabetes dietary self-management. *Diabetes Care* 1996; **19**: 835–842.

47. Glasgow RE, La Chance P, Toobert DJ, Brown J, Hampson SE, Riddle MC. Long term effects and costs of brief behavioral dietary intervention for patients with diabetes delivered from the medical office. *Patient Educ Couns* 1997; **32**: 175–184.

48. Riley KM, Glasgow RE, Eakin EG. Resources for health: A social–ecological intervention for supporting self-management of chronic conditions. *J Health Psychol* 2001; **6**: 693–705.

49. Glasgow RE, Strycker LA, Toobert DJ, Eakin EG. The Chronic Illness Resources Survey: A social–ecologic approach to assessing support for disease self-management. *J Behav Med* 2000; **23**: 559–583.

50. Piette JD, McPhee SJ, Weinberger M, Mah CA, Kraemer FB. Use of automated telephone disease management calls in an ethnically diverse sample of low-income patients with diabetes. *Diabetes Care* 1999; **22**: 1302–1309.

51. Piette JD, Weinberger M, Kraemer FB, McPhee SJ. The impact of automated calls with nurse follow-up on diabetes treatment outcomes in a Veterans Affairs health care system. *Diabetes Care* 2001; **24**: 202–208.

52. Litzelman DK, Slemenda CW, Langefeld CD *et al.* Reduction of lower extremity clinical abnormalities in patients with non-insulin-dependent diabetes mellitus: A randomized, controlled trial. *Ann Intern Med* 1993; **119**: 36–41.

53. Weinberger M, Kirkman MS, Samsa GP *et al.* A nurse-coordinated intervention for primary care patients with non-insulin-dependent mellitus: Impact on glycemic control and health-related quality of life. *J Gen Intern Med* 1995; **10**: 59–66.

54. Lichtenstein E, Glasgow RE, Lando HA, Ossip-Klein DJ, Boles SM. Telephone counseling for smoking cessation: Rationales and review of evidence. *Health Educ Res* 1996; **11**: 243–257.

55. Wasson J, Gaudette C, Whaley F, Sauvigne A, Baribeau P, Welch HG. Telephone care as a substitute for routine clinic follow-up. *JAMA* 1992; **267**: 1788–1793.

56. DCCT Research Group. The effect of intensive treatment of diabetes on the development and progression of long-term complications in insulin-dependent diabetes mellitus. *N Engl J Med* 1993; **329**: 977–986.

57. Fisher EB Jr, Arfken CL, Heins JM, Houston CA, Jeffe DB, Sykes RK. Acceptance of diabetes in adults. In Gochman DS (ed.), *Handbook of Health Behavior Research II: Provider Determinants*. New York: Plenum, 1997, pp 189–212.

58. Eastman RC, Siebert CW, Harris M, Gorden P. Clinical review: Implications of the Diabetes Control and Complications Trial. *J Clin Endocrinol Metab* 1993; **77**: 1105–1107.

59. Fisher EB Jr, Heins JM, Hiss RG *et al. Metabolic Control matters: Nationwide Translation of the Diabetes Control and Complications Trial: Analysis and Recommendations*, NIH

Publication No. 94-3773. Bethesda, MD: National Institute of Diabetes and Digestive and Kidney Diseases, 1994.

60. DeBusk RF, Miller NH, Superko HR. A case-management system for coronary risk factor modification after acute myocardial infarction. *Ann Intern Med* 1994; **120**: 721–729.
61. Bandura A. *Self-Efficacy: the Exercise of Control.* New York: Freeman, 1997.
62. Glasgow RE, Toobert DJ, Hampson SE, Noell JW. A brief office-based intervention to facilitate diabetes self-management. *Health Educ Res Theory Practice* 1995; **10**: 467–478.
63. Wagner EH, Grothaus LC, Sandhu N *et al.* Chronic care clinics for diabetes in primary care: A system-wide randomized trial. *Diabetes Care* 2001; **24**: 695–700.
64. Sadur CN, Moline N, Costa M *et al.* Diabetes management in a health maintenance organization: Efficacy of care management using cluster visits. *Diabetes Care* 1999; **22**: 2011–2017.
65. Lorig KR, Mazonson PD, Holman HR. Evidence suggesting that health education for self-management in patients with chronic arthritis has sustained health benefits while reducing health care costs. *Arthritis Rheum* 1993; **36**: 439–446.
66. Leveille SG, Wagner EH, Davis C *et al.* Preventing disability and managing chronic illness in frail older adults: A randomized trial of a community-based partnership with primary care. *JAGS* 1998; **46**: 1–9.
67. Lorig KR, Sobel DS, Stewart AL *et al.* Evidence suggesting that a chronic disease self-management program can improve health status while reducing hospitalization: A randomized trial. *Med Care* 1999; **37**: 5–14.
68. Skinner CS, Strecher VJ, Hospers H. Physicians' recommendations for mammography: Do tailored messages make a difference? *Am J Public Health* 1994; **84**: 43–49.
69. Gustafson DH, Hawkins R, Boberg E *et al.* Impact of a patient-centered, computer-based health information/support system. *Am J Prev Med* 1999; **16**: 1–9.
70. Anderson RM, Funnell MM, Barr PA, Dedrick RF, Davis WK. Learning to empower patients: Results of a professional education program for diabetes educators. *Diabetes Care* 1991; **14**: 584–590.
71. Anderson RM, Funnell MM, Butler PM, Arnold MS, Fitzgerald JT, Feste CC. Patient empowerment: Results of a randomized controlled trial. *Diabetes Care* 1995; **18**: 943–949.
72. Miller WR, Rollnick S. *Motivational Interviewing: Preparing People to Change Addictive Behavior.* New York: Guilford, 1991.
73. Wagner EH, Austin B, Von Korff M. Improving outcomes in chronic illness. *Manag Care Q* 1996; **4**: 12–25.
74. Wagner EH, Austin BT, Von Korff M. Organizing care for patients with chronic illness. *Milbank Q* 1996; **74**: 511–544.
75. Wagner EH, Glasgow RE, Davis C *et al.* Quality improvement in chronic illness care: A collaborative approach. *Joint Commission J Quality Improvement* 2001; **27**: 63–80.
76. McCulloch DK, Davis C, Austin BT, Wagner EH. Constructing a bridge across the quality chasm: A practical way to get healthier, happier patients, providers, and health care delivery systems. *Diabetes Spectrum* 2004; **17**: 92–96.
77. Institute for Healthcare Improvement. The Breakthrough Series: IHI's Collaborative Model for Achieving Breakthrough Improvement. *Diabetes Spectrum* 2004; **17**: 97–101.
78. Hupke C, Camp AW, Chaufournier R, Langley GJ, Little K. Transforming diabetes health care Part 2. Changing lives. *Diabetes Spectrum* 2004; **17**: 107–111.
79. Glasgow RE, Funnell MM, Bonomi AE, Davis C, Beckham V, Wagner EH. Self-management aspects of the improving chronic illness care Breakthrough Series: Implementation with diabetes and heart failure teams. *Ann Behav Med* 2002; **24**: 80–87.
80. Wagner EH, Austin BT, Davis C, Hindmarsh M, Schaefer J. Improving chronic illness care: Translating evidence into action. *Health Affairs* 2001; **20**: 64–78.

81. Glasgow RE, Davis CL, Funnell MM, Beck A. Implementing practical interventions to support chronic illness self-management in health care settings: Lessons learned and recommendations. *Joint Commission J Quality and Safety* 2003; **29**: 563–574.

82. Sallis JF, Owen N. Ecological models. In Glanz K, Lewis FM, Rimer BK (eds), *Health Behavior and Health Education: Theory, Research and Practice*. San Francisco, CA: Jossey-Bass, 1996, pp 403–424.

83. Stokols D. Establishing and maintaining healthy environments: Toward a social ecology of health promotion. *Am Psychol* 1992; **47**: 6–22.

84. Glasgow RE, McKay HG, Feil EG, Barrera M. The D-Net diabetes self-management program: Long-term implementation, outcomes, and generalization results. *Prev Med* 2003; **36**: 410–419.

85. Glasgow RE, Toobert DJ, Hampson SE, Strycker LA. Implementation, generalization, and long-term results of the 'Choosing Well' diabetes self-management intervention. *Patient Educ Couns* 2002; **48**: 115–122.

86. Schillinger D, Piette JD, Bindman A. Closing the loop: Missed opportunities in communicating with diabetes patients who have health literacy problems. *Arch Intern Med* 2003; **163**: 83–90.

87. Abrams DB, Orleans CT, Niaura RS, Goldstein MG, Prochaska JO, Velicer W. Integrating individual and public health perspectives for treatment of tobacco dependence under managed health care: A combined stepped care and matching model. *Ann Behav Med* 1996; **18**: 290–304.

88. Johnson SB. Compliance and control in insulin-dependent diabetes: Does behavior really make a difference? In Krasnegor NA, Epstein L, Johnson SB, Yaffe SJ (eds), *Developmental Aspects of Health Compliance Behavior*. Hillsdale, NJ: Erlbaum, 1993, pp 275–297.

89. Glasgow RE, McCaul KD, Schafer LC. Self-care behaviors and glycemic control in Type I diabetes. *J Chron Dis* 1987; **40**: 399–412.

90. Rost KM, Flavin KS, Schmidt LE, McGill JB. Self-care predictors of metabolic control in NIDDM patients. *Diabetes Care* 1990; **13**: 1111–1113.

91. Jenkins CD. An integrated behavioral medicine approach to improving care of patients with diabetes mellitus. *Behav Med* 1995; **21**: 53–65.

92. Kaplan RM. Behavior as the central outcome in health care. *Am Psychol* 1990; **45**: 1211–1220.

93. Glasgow RE, Osteen VL. Evaluating diabetes education: Are we measuring the most important outcomes? *Diabetes Care* 1992; **15**: 1423–1432.

94. Glasgow RE. Behavioral and psychosocial measures for diabetes care: What is important to assess? *Diabetes Spectrum* 1997; **10**: 12–17.

95. UK Prospective Diabetes Study Group. Intensive blood-glucose control with suphonylureas or insulin compared with conventional treatment and risk of complications in patients with type 2 diabetes (UKPDS 33). *Lancet* 1998; **352**: 837–853.

96. Hampson SE, Glasgow R, Toobert DJ. Personal models of diabetes and their relations to self-care activities. *Health Psychol* 1990; **9**: 632–646.

97. Hampson SE, Glasgow RE, Foster L. Personal models of diabetes among older adults: Relation to self-management and other variables. *Diabetes Educ* 1995; **21**: 300–307.

98. Glasgow RE, Ruggiero L, Eakin EG, Dryfoos J, Chobanian L. Quality of life and associated characteristics in a large diverse sample of adults with diabetes. *Diabetes Care* 1997; **20**: 562–567.

99. Rubin RR, Biermann J, Toohey B. *Psyching Out Diabetes: a Positive Approach to Your Negative Emotions*. Los Angeles: RGA, 1992.

100. Anderson LA, Jenkins CM. Educational innovations in diabetes: Where are we now? *Diabetes Spectrum* 1994; **7**: 89–124.

101. Mazze RS, Etzwiler DD, Strock E *et al*. Staged diabetes management. *Diabetes Care* 1994; **17**: 56–66.

102. Glasgow RE, Eakin EG. Issues in diabetes self-management. In Shumaker SA, Schron EB, Ockene JK, McBee WL (eds), *The Handbook of Health Behavior Change*. New York: Springer, 1998, pp. 435–461.

103. Anderson RM, Fitzgerald JT, Funnell MM *et al*. Evaluation of an activated patient diabetes education newsletter. *Diabetes Educ* 1994; **20**: 29–34.

104. Joyner L, McNeeley S, Kahn R. ADA's provider recognition program. *HMO Practice* 1997; **11**: 168–170.

105. Fiore MC. The new vital sign. Assessing and documenting smoking status (commentary). *JAMA* 1991; **266**: 3183–3184.

106. Haire-Joshu D, Glasgow RE, Tibbs TL. Smoking and diabetes. *Diabetes Care* 1999; **26**: S89–S90.

107. Orleans CT, Glynn TJ, Manley MW, Slade J. Minimal-contact quit smoking strategies for medical settings. In Orleans CT, Slade J (eds), *Nicotine Addiction: Principles and Management*. New York: Oxford University Press, 1993, pp 181–220.

108. Karoly P. Self-management in health-care and illness prevention. In Snyder CR, Forsyth DR (eds), *Handbook of Social and Clinical Psychology*. New York: Pergamon, 1991.

109. Karoly P. Goal systems: An organizing framework for clinical assessment and treatment planning. *Psychol Assessment* 1993; **5**: 273–290.

110. Hampson SE, Glasgow RE, Zeiss AM. Coping with osteoarthritis by older adults. *Arthritis Care Res* 1996; **9**: 133–141.

111. Bandura A. *Social Foundations of Thought and Action: a Social Cognitive Theory*. Englewood Cliffs, NJ: Prentice-Hall, 1986.

112. Nouwen A, Gingras J, Talbot F, Bouchard S. The development of an empirical psychosocial taxonomy for patients with diabetes. *Health Psychol* 1997; **16**: 263–271.

113. Irvine AA, Saunders JT, Blank MB, Carter WR. Validation of scale measuring environmental barriers to diabetes-regimen adherence. *Diabetes Care* 1990; **13**: 705–711.

114. Glasgow RE. Social–environmental factors in diabetes: Barriers to diabetes self-care. In Bradley C (ed.), *Handbook of Psychology and Diabetes Research and Practice*. Chur, Switzerland: Harwood, 1994, pp 335–349.

115. Glasgow RE, McCaul KD, Schafer LC. Barriers to regimen adherence among persons with insulin-dependent diabetes. *J Behav Med* 1986; **9**: 65–77.

116. Glasgow RE, Gillette C, Toobert D. Psychosocial barriers to diabetes self-management and quality of life. *Diabetes Spectrum* 2001; **14**: 33–41.

117. Beaven DW, Scott RS. The organisation of diabetes care. In Alberti KGMM, Krall LP (eds), *The Diabetes Annual/2*. New York: Elsevier, 1986, pp 39–48.

118. Funnell MM, Anderson RM. Changing office practice and health care systems to facilitate diabetes self-management. *Curr Diabetes Rep* 2003; **3**: 127–133.

119. National Committee for Quality Assurance (NCQA). *Diabetes Physician Recognition Program (DPRP) Frequently Asked Questions: Measures for Adult Patients.* http:www.ncqa.org/dprp/dprpfaz.htm#adultmeasures. 2002.

120. Kawachi I, Kennedy BP, Lochner K, Prothrow-Stith D. Social capital, income inequality, and mortality. *Am J Public Health* 1997; **87**: 1491–1498.

121. Kaplan RM. *The Hippocratic Predicament: Affordability, Access, and Accountability in American Health Care*. San Diego, CA: Academic, 1993.

122. Lamm RD. *The Brave New World of Health Care*. Golden, CO: Fulcrum, 2004.

123. Toobert DJ, Strycker LA, Glasgow RE, Bagdade JD. If you build it, will they come? Reach and adoption associated with a comprehensive lifestyle management program for women with type 2 diabetes. *Patient Educ Couns* 2002; **48**: 99–105.

124. Amthauer H, Gaglio B, Glasgow RE, King DK. Strategies and lessons learned in patient recruitment during a diabetes self-management program conducted in a primary care setting. *Diabetes Educ* 2003; **29**: 673–681.

125. Eakin EG, Bull SS, Glasgow RE, Mason M. Reaching those most in need: A review of diabetes self-management interventions in disadvantaged populations. *Diabetes Metab Res Rev* 2002; **18**: 26–35.

126. Green LW, Richard L, Potvin L. Ecological foundations of health promotion. *Am J Health Promo* 1996; **10**: 270–281.

127. McNabb WL. Adherence in diabetes: Can we define it and can we measure it? (commentary). *Diabetes Care* 1997; **20**: 215–218.

128. Strecher VJ, Kreuter M, Den Boer DJ, Kobrin S, Hospers HJ, Skinner CS. The effects of computer-tailored smoking cessation messages in family practice settings. *J Fam Pract* 1994; **39**: 262–268.

129. Brug J, Glanz K, Van Assema P, Kok G, van Breukelen GJ. The impact of computer-tailored feedback and iterative feedback on fat, fruit, and vegetable intake. *Health Educ Behav* 1998; **25**: 517–531.

130. Goodman RM, Steckler A. A model for the institutionalization of health promotion programs. *Family Community Health*. 1987; **11**: 63–78.

131. Santacroce SJ, Maccarelli LM, Grey M. Intervention fidelity. *Nurs Res* 2004; **53**: 63–66.

7

Psychological Group Interventions in Diabetes Care

T. Chas Skinner and Nicole van der Ven

The need for effective, well evaluated psychosocial interventions to assist people in dealing with the daily demands of diabetes has been urgently stressed in several reviews.[1-4] Especially now that treatment regimens are becoming more and more intensive, comprehensive behavioural changes are required.[5] Additional psycho-social support is called for to help people to make these changes, and to preserve and sustain their efforts with the goal of optimizing both glycaemic control and quality of life.[5,6] As the burden of diabetes rapidly increases,[7] there is a pressing need to deliver diabetes care in a more comprehensive and cost-effective manner. Delivering care in a group instead of in an individual format may be an effective way of doing this.

7.1 Psychosocial Group Interventions in Medical Illness

Group therapy has been used successfully for decades in the treatment of a wide variety of psychiatric disorders and psychological problems. In patients with chronic illnesses, group interventions have become popular as an adjunct to medical treatment.[8]

Groups for people with medical illnesses mostly address coping difficulties rather than frank psychopathology. In contrast to many groups for people with psychological disorders, participants usually have very different past experiences, personality styles and resources. Yet sharing the same medical condition provides them with ample common ground.

Psychology in Diabetes Care   Edited by Frank J. Snoek and T. Chas Skinner
© 2005 John Wiley & Sons, Ltd.

While long standing intrapersonal problems often require attention in an individual therapy, a group format may be preferred to address other aspects, e.g. providing information, training in behavioural skills and addressing inter-personal skills. Advantages of group over individual counselling include obtaining emotional support from people with similar experiences and being able to use the experiences of others as a model. Being part of a group, being understood and understanding others and being able to give and receive help strengthens the sense of belonging and enhances emotional well-being. While exploration of long standing intrapersonal problems may be better addressed individually, groups provide a richer learning environment to recognize inadequate interpersonal patterns and skills.

Group interventions may be conducted either with participants who have diverse problems and concerns or with people all sharing the same problem. People with medical illnesses have many concerns in common: understanding the diagnosis and prognosis of their disease, coping with treatment and side-effects, emerging medications and treatments, adjusting to changes in lifestyle and level of functioning, changes in mood and energy, interpersonal relationships and existential issues, including changes in self-image, evaluation of priorities and dying.[8] A self-management programme originally developed for people with arthritis, for example, was successfully transferred to groups with varying chronic conditions.[9]

The differing nature of chronic and/or life-threatening illnesses obviously also presents illness-specific concerns. For people with diabetes, there are a number of specific concerns that are evident in the literature. In type 1 diabetes, fear of hypoglycaemia is a common concern, which is evidenced by the extensive use of the fear of hypoglycaemia scale,[10] and common to both type 1 and type 2 diabetes is the burden of dietary inflexibility and restriction.[11,12] Added to these is dealing with the uncertainties concerning the development and progression of complications in the distant future,[8] and with type 2 diabetes the problems of lack of symptoms in the early stages and the resulting doubts about the seriousness of diabetes.[13]

Group interventions may be classified into different types along a continuum ranging from education, focussed on providing information and teaching practical skills, to psychotherapeutic groups. The most common therapeutic approach aimed at people with chronic illnesses can be located in between these poles; these are psycho-educational group interventions usually following a short, structured format in which lecture, practice and group discussion are combined, or 'coping skill trainings,' which mostly aim to increase an individual's coping repertoire with a few developing coping behaviours that are more productive for enhancing well-being and glycaemic controls. These programmes typically include training in problem solving, coping skills, cognitive restructuring and stress management. Here interventions commonly use methods based on cognitive–behavioural therapy (CBT), which is particularly suitable for the usually short and structured format (six to 10 meetings) of these groups.[14] CBT type approaches would also seem key to improving outcomes, as in a recent meta-analysis of psycho-educational interventions in type 2 diabetes the use of cognitive reframing techniques was predictive of better outcomes.[15]

7.2 Psychosocial Group Interventions in Diabetes

In diabetes care, group interventions have been employed to reach many different ends, ranging from self-management training to group psychotherapy. In reviews, a large proportion of interventions are group based.[16,17] Intuitively, group interventions appear to be an appropriate and cost-effective way to address psychosocial issues in diabetes care. There is however still a lack of systematic, quantitative evaluation of the effectiveness of psychosocial interventions in diabetes in general,[1,3] and there is little scientific evidence of the preferability of group over individual formats, with some one-off 1:1 interventions having a substantial sustained impact on diabetes outcomes.[18] Research on the effectiveness of diabetes education for people with type 2 diabetes however does indicate that group education is at least as effective as individual care[19] and may be more efficient and cost-effective.[20]

This chapter aims to provide an overview of the use and effectiveness of psychosocial group interventions in diabetes care. Because more and more behavioural techniques are being incorporated into diabetes education, the distinction between educational and other types of group is often difficult. We have focused on groups providing social and emotional support and coping skill training, excluding educational interventions strictly aimed at enhancing knowledge and practical skills. We did however incorporate coping-oriented modules incorporated into more comprehensive self-management interventions. A summary of the identified literature on group programmes can be found in Table 7.1.

The remainder of this chapter describes (1) psychological group interventions aimed at psychological problems complicating diabetes, (2) psychological group interventions dealing with complications of diabetes, (3) psycho-educational group interventions dealing with problems with hypoglycaemia and (4) coping-oriented group interventions aimed at assisting people in dealing with the daily demands of diabetes, aimed at improving behavioural and emotional coping. It concludes with remarks on future directions for group work, and evaluation of group interventions.

7.3 Psychological Group Interventions Aimed at Psychological Problems Complicating Diabetes

Similar to populations suffering from other chronic medical conditions, the prevalence of psychological disorders, especially anxiety and depression, is relatively high among people with diabetes, adults[21] as well as children and

Table 7.1 Summary of published studies of group programmes in diabetes care

Ref.	Sample characteristics	Intervention	Programme format	Moderator	Design and assessments	Positive effects
Children/adolescents						
57	$n = 108$ adolescents attending diabetes camp age 13–17	Stress-management training (identify sources of stress, relaxation, exercise, problem, solving, cognitive restructuring)	71 h daily meetings	Young adults with experience as camp medical staff	Pre–post, assessments at week 1 and 7	Coping strategies
58	$n = 120$ campers between 13 and 17 years (mean 14.9 years)	Assertiveness communication training (problem solving, negotiating skills), through information, sharing and games and role playing	7 daily classes	Young adults with experience as camp medical staff	Pre–post, assessments at week 1 and 7, and 3 months follow-up	Self-reported assertiveness $p < 0.001$
59	$n = 21$ adolescents with diabetes < 18 months, and their peers ($n = 21$) Mean age 13.1; duration of diabetes 8.4 months	Education listening skills, problem solving focussed on peer support, stress management. Games, exercises	4 weekly 2 h sessions	Psychologist	Pre–post, with assessments at week 1 and week 4	Improved diabetes knowledge. Peers: self-worth. Parents: diabetes-related conflict
60	$n = 23$ adolescents in need of psychosocial support Mean age 15.2 years, duration of diabetes 4.6 years, HbA1c 10.6	Aims: provide social network, identify stressful issues, develop coping strategies, through group discussion, practicing (role-playing, field trips)	8 bimonthly 2 h meetings		Wait list controlled, with assessments before session 1/after session 8	Psychological functioning

61	$n = 21$ attenders of diabetes camp, aged between 13 and 18. Mean age 14.9 years, HbA1c 12.6; 46% female	I: social learning exercises to improve social skills C: diabetes education	Daily, 3 weeks (15 sessions)	Experts in diabetes care (endocrinologist, ophthalmologist, podiatrist)	Controlled, with assessments at first and final day, and at 4 months follow-up	Glycaemic control
63	$n = 11$ children with inadequate social skills. Age 9–12	Social skills training (modelling, role play) C: no treatment	10 sessions of 45 min twice a week	Experimenter (?)	Controlled pre–post with untreated control group Assessments at baseline, post-treatment, and 1 and 6 weeks follow-up	Coping with stressful diabetes-related social situations
65,66	$n = 65$ adolescents initiating intensive insulin therapy (IIT). Mean age 15.8 years; duration of diabetes 7.6 years; HbA1c 8.9%; 56% female	I: IIT with coping skills training (CST): problem solving, social skills, and cognitive behaviour modification through role play and modeling C: IIT	IIT: monthly visit, frequent telephone contact. CST: 4–8 weekly 1½ h sessions	Nurse specialized in diabetes and paediatric psychiatry	RCT, assessments at baseline, and 3, 6, 12 months follow-up	Improvements in HbA1c, self-efficacy, coping, QoL (3, 6, 12 months)
67	$n = 37$ adolescents with type 1 diabetes. Age 11–18. Mean age 13.4 years; duration of diabetes 4.5 years; 53% female	I: behavioural intervention (meal planning, self-monitoring of blood glucose, blood glucose discrimination training, stress management, cognitive restructuring, social skill training and problem solving. C: standard medical care	8 sessions (+ two assessments, and two with parents)	Psychologist	Non-randomized controlled, assessments at baseline, post-intervention and 12 months follow-up	Knowledge, self-care behaviours, psychosocial variables

Continues

Table 7.1 (*Continued*)

Ref.	Sample characteristics	Intervention	Programme format	Moderator	Design and assessments	Positive effects
68	$n = 21$ adolescents with HbA1c > 8.5%. Age 11–17, duration DM 6.2 years, 72% female, HbA1c 10.2%	I: motivational interviewing and solution-focussed therapy, including CBT C: those who refused to participate	6 weekly sessions	?	Non-randomized controlled. Assessments: HbA1c at baseline, 3, 6, 12 months follow-up. Psychological variable baseline, 6 months follow-up	HbA1c (6 months)
Adults						
69	$n = 9$ young women with adherence problems. Age 20–36	Stress management, assertiveness training, cognitive restructuring, dealing with criticism and anger, dealing with medical staff	12 weekly 3 h sessions	social worker	Pre–post	Self-reported self-care behaviours, self-confidence
70,71	$n = 165$, mean age 47 years, 42% female, 38% type 1 DM, 63% taking insulin; HbA1c 11.5	CBT-based coping skill training added to diabetes education programme. Identifying regimen barriers, generating/evaluating solutions, modifying dysfunctional cognitions, relapse prevention	2 sessions, a total of 2½ h	Social worker and mental health counsellor	Pre–post, with assessments at baseline, post-intervention and 6 months follow-up	6 months: emotional well-being, HbA1c, increased SMBG, reduced binge-eating. 12 months: self-esteem, anxiety, DM knowledge, self-efficacy

	Participants	Intervention	Duration	Provider	Design	Outcomes
72	n = 83 participants of inpatient teaching programme with inadequate glycaemic control. Mean age 35, HbA1c 8.1, 41% female	Psychosocial modules on individual goal-setting, group discussion on motivational/emotional aspects (acceptance, coping) incorporated in 5 day inpatient training and teaching programme	2 sessions of 2½ h		Pre-post, assessments at baseline and mean follow-up of 17.5 months	Self-efficacy, relationship with doctor, less externally controlled, reduced severe hypoglycaemia
73	n = 64, mean age 50, 54% using insulin	Empowerment programme: goal setting, problem-solving skills, emotional coping, stress management, obtaining social support, motivation. Introduction of key concepts, self-assessments, worksheets during and in between sessions, group discussion	6 weekly sessions	Diabetes educator	Waiting list controlled, partially randomized	Quality of life, attitude towards dm, HbA1c, self-efficacy
74	n = 73 type 2 patients with HbA1c > 8.5%, up to 60 years. C: n = 35	Goal setting, problem solving, coping with diabetes, coping with daily stress, seeking social support and staying motivated. Introduction of a topic, followed by group discussion, practical exercises and planning activities for in-between sessions.	6 weekly 90 min meetings	6 groups by psychologist, 2 groups by team of psychologist and diabetologist	Quasi experimental controlled study. Assessments: baseline, post-intervention, 3, 6, 12 months	Psychological and social aspects of quality of life, HbA1c (3, 6 months)

Continues

Table 7.1 (*Continued*)

Ref.	Sample characteristics	Intervention	Programme format	Moderator	Design and assessments	Positive effects
75	$n = 19$ type 2 patients classified as stress having negative impact on HbA1c. Mean age 59.8, 53% female, 84% oral medication, 16% diet; duration of DM 6.4 years, HbA1c 10.7	CBT stress-management programme. Training in progressive muscle relaxation, cognitive coping skills, problem-solving skills, homework assignments	6 weekly 90 min sessions	Therapist	Pre–post, waiting list controlled	Stress, anxiety
76	$n = 24$ people with diabetes with self-management problems. Mean age 43.5, duration DM 11.7 years, 42% female	Pro-active coping programme, emphasizing goal-setting, planning of behaviour. Maintaining good physical condition; preventing exacerbation (symptom recognition, adequate action); coping with negative emotions (anger, anxiety, relaxation); seeking social support. Discussion of homework, introduction of a topic, individual goal setting, group discussion. Acting on behavioural plan and registering goal attainment in between sessions	5 bi-weekly 2 h sessions	Diabetes nurse specialist		Not available yet

77	n = 24 type 1 dm with HbA1c > 8%. Mean age 35.2. 63% female, HbA1c 9.3%	Cognitive Behavioural Group Training (CBGT). Cognitive restructuring; stress management; worries about complications and the future; social relationships. Discussion of homework, introduction of a topic, group discussion and exercises. Cognitive and behavioural homework assignments.	4 weekly 90 min sessions	Psychologist and diabetes nurse specialist	Uncontrolled pilot study	HbA1c
78	n = 74 type 1 diabetic patients, 68% female; mean age 31.2 years; HbA1c 9.8	I: CBT-based intervention (cognitive restructuring, relaxation) C: cholesterol education	I: 8 weekly sessions	Psychologist	RCT	I+C: adherence, HbA1c I: Qol
79	n = 88 type 1 dm with HbA1c > 8%. Mean age 37.8 year, duration dm 18.0 year, 59% female, HbA1c 8.9%	I: CBGT with additional individual goal-setting and session on 'diabetes as teamwork' C: BGAT	6 weekly 90 min sessions	Psychologist and diabetes nurse specialist	RCT with 3 month run-in period. Assessments: baseline, pre-intervention, 3, 6, 12 months follow-up	I+C: diabetes-related emotional distress (PAID), depressive symptoms, diabetes-specific self-efficacy

adolescents.[22] While anxiety and depression obviously have an important impact on coping with diabetes in children and adolescents, their association with metabolic control in the adolescent population has not been clearly established yet.[22] In adults with diabetes, depression may result in deterioration of physical and emotional well-being and disruption of self-care routines. Depressive symptoms have been shown to be associated with poor medical outcomes.[23]

Treatment of psychological disorders (psychotherapeutical and/or pharmacological) mainly takes place in individual therapy; there are no examples of group treatment for depression in diabetes.

A systematic review shows that generalized anxiety disorder (GAD), the most prevalent of the anxiety disorders, also occurs more frequently among people with diabetes (14 per cent as opposed to three to four per cent observed in US community studies).[24] Anxiety disorders appear to be associated with hyperglycaemia only when established through a diagnostic interview, and not when anxiety is self-reported.[25] This suggests that treatment of anxiety may improve glycaemic control. Similar to treatment of depression, however, anxiety-related psychological disorders are mostly treated in an individual format.

Whether elevated levels of distress are attributable to the psychological stress of self-management, to fears of complications or hypoglycaemia or to diabetes-related abnormalities in neurohormonal/neurotransmitter function still needs to be established in longitudinal studies.[24] Nevertheless, the notion that glycaemic control is affected by psychological stress has been established both in research and in the subjective experience of people with diabetes. It has been hypothesized that stress may cause poor glycaemia either directly, through the hyperglycaemic effect of stress hormones, or indirectly, by disruption of self-care routines.[2] Interventions aimed at modifying the behavioural effects of stress are often incorporated into more comprehensive coping-skill programmes, to be discussed later in this chapter.

Methods to help patients reduce physiological arousal caused by stress directly include biofeedback assisted relaxation training (BART) and progressive muscle relaxation (PMR), usually in a time-intensive individual format. There are some examples however of these methods applied in a group setting.

Surwit *et al.*[26] evaluated the efficacy and feasibility of a cost-effective outpatient group programme for stress management training in a randomized, controlled trial. Individuals with type 2 diabetes ($n = 108$; not on insulin; mean age 57.3 ± 10.7 years; mean A1c 7.9 ± 1.8 per cent) were randomized to either a control group ($n = 48$) receiving five weekly group sessions of diabetes education, or the experimental group ($n = 60$), attending five sessions of stress management training, involving PMR, instruction in stress-reducing cognitive and behavioural skills (identifying stressors, guided imagery, thought stopping) and education on health consequences of stress. Participants practiced PMR between sessions using audiotapes. Throughout 6 months, A1c results improved equally in both groups. At 12-month follow-up, improvements were sustained in the stress management group only and resulted in a significant 0.5 per cent reduction in A1c results. The intervention did not have any effect on perceived stress, anxiety or general psychological health. Researchers did not find evidence to support the hypothesis that stress management is of greater benefit to subjects with higher levels of anxiety.

In an earlier small, controlled study on stress management training for groups of type 2 diabetic patients ($n = 22$; mean age 61.0 ± 10.2 years; mean A1c 11.0 ± 1.9 per cent), participants were randomized to relaxation training or routine medical care.[27] In six weekly 1 hour sessions, PMR, imagery and group discussion of stressful life events were addressed. At four-month follow-up, training did not have any effect on glycaemic control, generalized distress, anxiety or daily hassles. Higher levels of anxiety and distress at baseline were associated with less improvement in glucose tolerance in the intervention group.

These short term interventions aimed at reducing physiological arousal in older patients were not successful in modifying psychological variables related to stress and had mixed effects on glycaemic control. These findings suggest that highly anxious individuals might respond better to individually administered interventions.[27]

The impact of a stress management and relaxation programme on glycaemic control and mood was evaluated in a randomized, waiting list-controlled study.[28] Participants were people with type 1 diabetes who perceived themselves as having stress-related difficulties in their daily life and in the management of their diabetes ($n = 36$; mean age 40.8 ± 12.4 years; mean A1c 7.3 ± 1.4 per cent mean duration of diabetes 10.5 years; 61 per cent female). The programme consisted of 14 2 h group meetings, in which instruction in stress and stress management, muscle relaxation, mental imaging and mental goal-setting were practiced. Improvements in relaxation and tension were largest for those with poorest scores at baseline. No improvements in mood or HbA1c were reported, probably due to already neutral to positive mood states and satisfactory glycaemic control at the start of the study.

One issue that should be considered when evaluating the research and clinical utilization of stress-management programmes is that not everyone is stress reactive. Some individuals seem to show marked elevations in blood glucose levels in relation to stress. However, this would not appear to be true for everyone, with some individuals showing no obvious association between blood glucose levels and stress levels.[29,30] These studies also suggest that people with diabetes are fairly good at identifying whether they are stress reactive in terms of blood glucose levels, and Polonsky[31] has suggested a relatively simple method for establishing stress reactivity. Although the relative proportions of stress-reactive individuals is not known, current data would not suggest this is the majority of individuals with diabetes, but no large population data is yet available to inform this issue.

Although there has been much debate, it would appear that although anorexia and bulimia seem to be marginally more prevalent in people with type 1 diabetes the diagnostic label 'eating disorders not otherwise specified' (EDNOS) appears to be twice as common among girls and young women with diabetes.[32] The eating disorders identified, meeting DSM-IV criteria as well as subthreshold disorders, were associated with body dissatisfaction, dietary restriction, insulin omission and other forms of purging, and were associated with poor glycaemic control and chronic complications. The distinctive features of diabetes treatment that may increase the risk (e.g. dietary restraints, inherent weight gain) and the potential serious consequences (poor glycaemic control and complications) of eating disorders require early detection and treatment. These factors have led to the development of several group interventions for women with diabetes.

In a small study ($n = 14$), a six-session group psycho-educational programme for women with type 1 diabetes and subclinical eating disorders was no more successful than the waiting-list control condition. Both groups showed improved psychological functioning but no changes in metabolic control, treatment adherence or eating disorder symptomatology.[33]

In a randomized controlled trial, Olmsted et al.[34] evaluated the effects of a brief intervention for young women with type 1 diabetes and disordered eating attitudes and behaviour. Participants ($n = 85$, age 12–20 years, mean A1c 9.1 ± 1.5 per cent) with elevated scores on the Eating Disorder Inventory were randomized to the intervention or treatment as usual. Delivered in a didactic style, the programme was not designed for in-depth discussion of personal information. Six 90 minute sessions provided oral and written didactic information on eating problems, how to control symptoms of disturbed eating and concerns about body image, with emphasis on the relationship between disordered eating and diabetes. Parents participated in identically structured but separate groups. Sessions were conducted by one professional with expertise in eating disorders and one familiar with adolescent diabetes. The programme resulted in a reduction of disturbed eating attitudes, which was maintained at six-month follow-up, but no reduction of insulin omission or A1c results.

Kenardy et al.[35] evaluated the effects of cognitive behavioural group therapy (CBGT) on binge eating. Women with type 2 diabetes ($n = 34$; mean age 54.88 ± 10.47 years; mean A1c 7.46 ± 1.50 per cent; 56 per cent diet only, 38 per cent oral medication, six per cent insulin) were randomized to 10 weekly sessions of CBGT ($n = 17$) or non-prescriptive therapy (NPT, $n = 17$) focussing on acceptance of negative affect. Both interventions improved binge eating, mood, eating-related beliefs and weight equally, but neither had any effect on glycaemic control. CBGT participants remaining abstinent of bingeing at the end of treatment maintained their success at three-month follow-up, whereas NPT participants showed significant relapse. Bingeing seems a worthwhile target, in that reduction of bingeing frequency, controlling for reduction of body mass index, was associated with improvement in A1c results. Participants with more frequent binge episodes showed the least improvement, suggesting they need longer or more intensive treatment.

Although attitudes were modified, the short term interventions using an educational approach were not successful in changing actual behaviour. Eating disorders seem to require interventions with more opportunity for interaction, as modelled in the Kenardy study.[35] The behavioural focus of CBGT seems useful in helping to maintain behavioural changes in the longer term.

7.4 Psychological Group Interventions Dealing with Complications of Diabetes

The diagnosis of diabetes itself is regarded as an emotionally upsetting event for many – if not all – people with diabetes. Several group interventions have been described, designed to help people through the emotional turmoil they may face when confronted with a diagnosis of diabetes. An early report describes positive effects of a crisis intervention clinic with discussion groups available for parents and children.[36] The unique setting of this clinic, however, makes it hard to single out the added value of the group meetings. A more recent study[37] developed a programme to help patients with type 1 diabetes reduce distress at disease onset and to achieve better future adaptation. Participants were enrolled in a prospective randomized controlled trial at the time of diagnosis ($n = 23$; 61 per cent female; mean age 24.52 ± 4.62 years; mean HbA1c 10.33 ± 1.71 per cent). They all received standard intensive treatment and diabetes education, with ($n = 10$) or without ($n = 13$) the distress reduction programme. Twenty-five weekly meetings lasting 90 minutes each were led by a psychotherapist, who brought up the following topics: expression of grief and anxiety about the loss of health; impact on social and family life; anxiety about hypo- and hyperglycaemia and late complications; and unconscious personality patterns (denial, frustration, aggression). The programme had a positive impact on depression, anxious coping style and denial three months after treatment. However, even this intervention offering extensive face-to-face contact was not successful in maintaining benefits in the longer term.

In research on diabetes-related emotional distress, 'Worrying about the future and the possibility of serious complications' is consistently rated as most distressful by people with type 1 as well as type 2 diabetes, followed by 'Feelings of guilt and anxiety when you get off track with your diabetes management'.[38] Complications patients may face later in the disease may require renewed adaptation and the reestablishment of emotional equilibrium.

People with diabetes do not seem to underestimate the seriousness of diabetes and its consequences. When compared with DCCT data, patients appear to overestimate their risk for major complications and the benefits of intensive treatment in reducing their risks.[39] A similar result has also been found for people with type 2 diabetes, who overestimated their risk for developing CHD.[40] This may be beneficial, when perception of vulnerability to illness and efficacy of therapy motivates patients to become actively involved in self-management of diabetes. However, if individuals do not believe in the efficacy of treatment strategies, or feel unable to implement them, this may result in high levels of fear, causing feelings of helplessness and denial.

For visually impaired people with diabetes, several group interventions have been described. An early study[41] offered an account of a short term (seven weekly sessions) therapy group with four visually impaired patients, but contained only descriptive outcomes. Caditz[42] has also described a support group for people with diabetes and visual impairment. The aims of the group were to give information about diabetes and visual impairment and to increase independence and self-esteem by providing emotional support. Groups of participants between the ages of 20 and 80 years met for 2 hours a week for 10–12 weeks. The meetings resulted in improved knowledge and use of visual aids, and group support helped participants emphasize the positives of their situation.

Aims of another combined educational/support group were to improve independence, self-esteem and glycaemic control in blind people ($n = 29$) with type 1 or type 2 diabetes.[43] A multidisciplinary team delivered three sessions a week for 12 weeks, focusing on diabetes self-management skills for the visually impaired, monitored exercise and group support. The programme was successful in improving glycaemic control, exercise tolerance and psychosocial indices.

Fear of complications is a major concern for many patients, and may result in avoidance and neglect of diabetes care in some patients and in extreme concern and overreaction to diabetes in others. Zettler et al.[44] developed a behavioural group programme teaching participants with type 1 diabetes strategies to cope with complications. The aim of the intervention was to reduce anxiety and avoidance behaviour, encourage adherence and prepare patients for crises. Patients who reported elevated levels of anxiety on a screening instrument ($n = 17$; 65 per cent female; 18 per cent on insulin; mean age 58.3 ± 9.8 years; mean A1c 9.4 ± 1.6 per cent), participated in an uncontrolled study. A psychologist delivered the programme, consisting of cognitive behavioural strategies (exposure in imagination, relaxation training, analysis of dysfunctional health beliefs) to small groups of four to six patients. The programme consisted of six 1.5 hour sessions, with an additional three-month follow-up session to report progress and discuss modification of goals and coping strategies. The majority of participants already had complications. At three months, results showed a reduction of fear and enhanced acceptance of the disease.

Recent studies show that diabetic peripheral neuropathy, ultimately resulting in foot ulceration and amputation, is associated with worsened physical and psychosocial functioning.[45,46] Furthermore, recent reviews indicate that the best that pharmacological or alternative analgesic approaches can achieve is moderate pain relief.[47] Therefore, it is not surprising that poor well-being is a consequence of pessimistic beliefs (e.g. perceived lack of control, self-blame) and impaired physical and social functioning. Therefore, providing individuals with the skills necessary to cope with painful neuropathy would seem to be an obvious need for this population. Unfortunately, there have been no published interventions aimed at the understanding of these complications and their emotional responses.[45] Psychological interventions are needed to assist people to deal with negative emotional responses in a constructive, helpful way by providing them with emotional and behavioural tools to do so.

7.5   Psychological Group Interventions Dealing with Hypoglycaemia

With intensification of insulin treatment, hypoglycaemic episodes have become more prevalent. Especially severe hypoglycaemic episodes, requiring the assistance of others to be alleviated, can be threatening physically and emotionally. Over the past two decades, a behavioural group programme called Blood Glucose Awareness Training (BGAT) has been developed and evaluated to assist patients with type 1 diabetes to recognize, predict, avoid and treat hypo- and hyperglycaemic episodes more effectively.

The most recent version of BGAT consists of a training manual and eight weekly group meetings involving behavioural techniques (e.g. self-monitoring, direct feedback, active homework exercises). Four classes deal with recognizing symptoms of high and low blood glucose (e.g. physical symptoms of hormonal counter-regulation, signs of neuroglycopenia, mood swings) and psychological factors influencing accurate detection and interpretation (e.g. attention, distraction, competing explanations, denial). The latter part of BGAT provides participants with information on food, exercise, and insulin to modify treatment decisions that may contribute to glucose dysregulation.[48]

Several studies have confirmed the effectiveness of BGAT in improving detection of hypoglycaemia and hyperglycaemia. A multicentre study ($n = 79$; 64 per cent female; mean age 38.2 ± 9.0 years; mean A1c 10.3 ± 2.1 per cent) showed BGAT was most effective among patients with reduced hypoglycaemic awareness.[49] Subjects maintained improved detection and reduced frequency of high and low blood glucose levels at 12-month follow-up and had fewer episodes of diabetic ketoacidosis and severe hypoglycaemia. Additionally, BGAT had beneficial effects on psychological functioning.[50]

A randomized, controlled study with type 1 diabetic patients enrolled in an outpatient intensive diabetes treatment programme showed improved glycaemic control in BGAT and control groups. However, BGAT was successful in preserving protective counter-regulatory responses to hypoglycaemia, thus suggesting that BGAT is a useful tool to decrease blunting of counter-regulation associated with improved glycaemic control.[51]

A Dutch study found no differences between the effect of BGAT delivered to groups compared with individual training. Overall results showed no positive effects of BGAT. This may be because of the use of a shortened version of BGAT or because of a small sample size.[52]

BGAT improved the ability to detect high and low blood glucose in a small group of adolescents when compared with untreated control subjects. Participants' performance after training, however, still remained poorer than that of adults.[53] No controlled studies of BGAT for younger children are available. Based on this former work, a group intervention was recently developed in Germany to assist people with type 1 diabetes to improve self-management associated with hypoglycaemia, improve their awareness of hypoglycaemia and prevent problems associated with hypoglycaemia.[54] In three 2 hour group sessions delivered by a psychologist, attitudes towards hypoglycaemia are discussed, participants learn about hypoglycaemia (individual symptoms, symptom perception, causes of reduced awareness) and insulin therapy, they talk about how to deal with hypoglcyaemia in daily life and they learn techniques for self-monitoring (e.g. hypoglycaemia diaries), with the optional support of hand-held computers. The programme was evaluated in people with type 1 diabetes admitted to hospital for two weeks to participate in group education for initiation of CSII ($n = 105$, 37.0 years, 61 per cent female, 16.4 years dm, HbA1c 7.0 per cent). The control group consisted of CSII group participants attending conventional individual education on hypoglycaemia (two 45 min sessions with a psychologist; $n = 102$, 34.3 years, 60 per cent female, 16.2 years dm, HbA1c 7.0 per cent) (data on evaluation in preparation, Kubiak).

7.6   Groups Dealing with the Daily Demands of Diabetes

Coping with the daily demands of diabetes is hard for many, if not all, people with diabetes. Various group interventions attempt to help patients cope more effectively with the daily hassles of diabetes. These coping-oriented group interventions typically consist of problem-solving and/or social skill training and use cognitive and behavioural strategies.

In children and adolescents, training in coping skills is usually aimed at improving assertiveness and social skills. The short and structured nature of these interventions seems to have positive effects on attendance[55] and assertiveness.[56]

Two uncontrolled studies involving adolescents in diabetes camp settings added a 'life skill' component to diabetes education.[57,58] One study[57] evaluated the effect of stress-management training in campers who received 1 hour of training each day for a week. Campers learned to identify sources of stress and to use stress-management techniques (relaxation, imagery, exercise, problem solving, identification and modification of negative automatic thoughts in stressful situations). After camp, participants used more adaptive coping strategies.[57] A similar training in assertive communication skills[58] resulted in improvement of self-reported assertiveness.

To enhance peer support, Greco et al.[59] offered groups providing both education and support to adolescents with a recent diagnosis of type 1 diabetes and their best friends. Goal was to integrate peers into diabetes care in a healthy, adaptive manner. Groups of adolescent–peer pairs met for four weekly 2 hour sessions delivered by a psychologist. Sessions focussed on education, listening skills, problem solving (with a focus on potential support by peers) and stress management. Topics were practiced through games, exercises and homework assignments.

Both adolescents with diabetes and their peers showed an increase in knowledge after the intervention. Actual support, which was already high at baseline, did not improve. Self-worth improved in peers, which may have reflected the significance of being able to provide support. Parents reported a decrease in diabetes-related conflict. Attendance in this study was excellent, which underscores the social validity of including peers in interventions for adolescents. In a waiting-list-controlled study by Marrero et al.[60] group discussion on diabetes-related issues perceived as stressful, collective identification of coping strategies and practice through role-play and exercise were used to provide adolescents with supportive social networks to help them cope more effectively with crises. This long-term group (2 hour semi-monthly meetings for eight months) included adolescents identified as potentially benefiting from psychosocial support but not requiring psychotherapy. Participants showed better psychological functioning when compared with control subjects.

Adolescents with type 1 diabetes attending a three-week summer school were randomized to daily social learning exercises to improve social skills and the ability to resist peer pressure or a control group spending an equal amount of time learning medical facts about diabetes. At four-month follow-up, glycaemic control in the social skills group was better than that of control subjects.[61] Results were replicated by Massouh et al.[62]

For children identified as having inadequate social skills, 10 sessions of specific training using modeling and role playing resulted in improved coping abilities but not in improved HbA1c results.[63]

In adolescents with a history of poor adherence and control, a 13-session training in stress management involving cognitive restructuring, assertive communication, problem solving, role playing and discussion was successful in reducing diabetes-specific distress when compared with an untreated control group, but left glycaemic control, adherence, and coping behaviour unchanged.[64]

A randomized, controlled study evaluated the effects of coping skill training (CST).[65] This is a programme aimed to increase participants' sense of competence and mastery by retraining non-constructive coping styles and forming more positive patterns of behaviour in adolescents initiating intensive insulin therapy. Adolescents were randomized to intensive management with or without CST. Intensive management included monthly outpatient visits and frequent telephone contacts. For four to eight weekly sessions of 60–90 minutes each, groups of two to three patients met with a nurse practitioner experienced in diabetes and paediatric psychiatry. They practiced problem solving, social skills and cognitive behaviour modification through role playing and modelling, using scenarios of difficult diabetes-related situations. At three months, CST participants showed greater improvement in A1c, self-efficacy, coping and quality of life than did control subjects. Positive effects were maintained at six- and 12-month follow-up.[66] In female participants, CST resulted in decreased weight gain and less hypoglycaemia.

A non-randomized behavioural programme aimed at improving treatment adherence and stress management in adolescents also had positive effects on psychosocial variables that were maintained at 12-month follow-up.[67] Adolescents with type 1 diabetes participated in a behavioural intervention or continued to receive standard medical care. The intervention group attended 12 sessions (including two sessions for assessment and two with their parents). During the remaining eight sessions, participants received instruction and practice in meal planning, self-monitoring of blood glucose, blood glucose discrimination training, stress management, cognitive restructuring, social skill training and problem solving.

In a non-randomized controlled pilot study, a group intervention based on motivational solution-focussed therapy was delivered to adolescents (11–17 years) to help them improve their poor glycaemic control (HbA1c > 8.5).[68] The intervention was based on motivational interviewing and solution-focussed therapy, including elements of CBT. Participants attended six weekly sessions; control subjects were randomly selected from those refusing to participate. The intervention proved effective in improving HbA1c at 6 months follow-up (10.2 to 8.7 per cent, $p < 0.05$; controls 9.8 per cent). These findings should however be interpreted with caution: reach of the intervention seems low with only 21 of 126 (17 per cent) eligible patients willing to participate. The use of patients refusing the intervention as controls also seems problematic: it remains unclear whether improvements should be attributed to the intervention or simply to motivation to change.

Coping-oriented group interventions have also been found to benefit adults. A 12-session programme for young women selected on the basis of non-adherence successfully improved self-reported self-management behaviours and self-confidence.[69] However, the number of participants in this study was very small ($n = 9$).

Some studies have evaluated adding one or more sessions of coping skills training to an education programme. Rubin et al.[70] added to an outpatient education programme two sessions of diabetes-specific coping skills training based on a cognitive behavioural approach. This additional training included identifying individual regimen barriers, generating and evaluating potential solutions, identifying and modifying dysfunctional thinking patterns and learning strategies to prevent relapse. Participants showed improved emotional well-being and A1c, increased frequency of glucose monitoring and decreased bingeing six months after the intervention. Positive effects on self-esteem, anxiety, diabetes knowledge and self-efficacy were maintained at 12-month follow-up.[71]

Bott et al.[72] included psychosocial modules in a five-day inpatient training and teaching programme for patients with type 1 diabetes who were not in adequate glycaemic control. Beyond the education component, patients attended two sessions of group discussions on individual goal setting and motivational and emotional aspects such as acceptance and coping strategies. At follow-up, A1c remained constant, whereas severe hypoglycaemia decreased. Participants reported feeling less externally controlled and reported improvements in self-efficacy and their relationships with their doctor.

Empowerment is another approach to improving coping, problem solving and motivation. A study by Anderson et al.[73] used a partially randomized, waiting-list controlled design to evaluate the effects of a patient empowerment programme. Patients participated in six weekly sessions focusing on improvement in goal setting, problem-solving skills, emotional coping, stress management, obtaining social support and motivation. Each session contained a brief presentation of key concepts, individual self-assessment, planning worksheets during and between sessions and group discussion. A total of 64 patients (of which 46 were randomly assigned and 18 not randomized) participated. Results show modest improvements in the perceived impact of diabetes on quality of life, decline in negative attitude towards living with diabetes, a reduction in A1c results and improvement of self-efficacy specifically related to the programme content.

In a recent controlled study, an empowerment-based group intervention was delivered to people with type 2 diabetes in poor glycaemic control (HbA1c > 8.5 per cent).[74]

The programme consisted of six weekly small group meetings, in which the following topics were covered: goal setting, problem solving, coping with diabetes, coping with daily stress, seeking social support and staying motivated. In each session, a short introduction of the topic was followed by group discussion, practical exercises and planning activities for period in between sessions. Six groups were moderated by a psychologist and two by a team of a psychologist and diabetologist.

The most common difficulties reported by participants were problems arising from everyday life. The most common benefit of the intervention reported was experiencing support. Results show that psychological as well as social aspects of quality of life were improved after the intervention. HbA1c was reduced until six months follow-up (9.7 at baseline to 9.3 directly after and 8.9 and 9.0 at three and six months respectively).

Looking at the reach of the intervention in this study, it is of interest that only 34 of the 173 potential participants interviewed (20 per cent) were regular attenders of the meetings.

Henry et al.[75] evaluated the efficacy of a combined cognitive–behavioural stress management programme in patients with type 2 diabetes whose physicians assessed that stress was subjectively affecting blood glucose levels. The programme aimed to reduce stress and improve glycaemic control. Patients were randomly allocated to the intervention or waiting list. Participants attended six weekly small group sessions of 1.5 hours delivered by a therapist. They received training in progressive muscle relaxation, cognitive coping skills and problem-solving skills and homework assignments that fostered practicing these skills. The programme had positive effects on self-reported stress and anxiety but did not affect A1c results or fasting blood glucose levels.

A short intervention aimed at improving self-management was developed for people with various chronic diseases, experiencing some failure in self-managing their disease.[76] Self-management problems were defined as shown by medical measures, symptoms, no-show at the clinic, ER visits or hospital admission. In line with the work of Lorig et al.,[9] the programme followed a general model but was provided to disease-homogeneous groups of patients. The programme was based on proactive coping, emphasizing goal-setting and the planning of behaviour. Five biweekly group sessions of 2 h were facilitated by specialized nurses. In the first two sessions, which were tailored to the needs of specific diseases, the topics of maintaining a good physical condition and preventing exacerbation (recognition of symptoms; taking adequate action) were covered. Sessions 3 and 4 dealt with coping with negative emotions in relation to being chronically ill (anger, irritation, anxiety, relaxation) and giving and seeking social support. The fifth session was delivered after four weeks to maintain behavioural changes. Each session followed the format of discussing homework, introduction of a theme, group discussion, individual goal setting and discussion. In between sessions, participants were supposed to act on their plans and keep a diary of goal attainment. No data on the effectiveness of this intervention has been provided yet. Evaluation of content shows that most participants were positive about the intervention; people with diabetes however did not rate the programme as high as patients with other medical conditions.

In two recent studies,[77,78] the utility of short, structured, well described group interventions based on principles of cognitive behavioural therapy was tested in groups of type 1 diabetic patients in long term poor glycaemic control. Snoek et al.[77] reported on a pilot study on the feasibility and efficacy of a CBGT program for patients with type 1 diabetes in persistent poor glycaemic control. The programme aimed to assist patients in overcoming negative beliefs and attitudes toward diabetes and achieving better glycaemic control without compromising emotional well-being. Twenty-four patients participated in four weekly sessions of 1.5 hours each delivered by a diabetes nurse specialist and a psychologist to small groups (six to eight patients). Each session addressed a different topic: the cognitive behavioural model of diabetes; stress and diabetes; living with the future (worries about complications) and social relationships. Training focused on cognitive restructuring, stress-management techniques and behavioural strategies (cueing, self-monitoring). CBGT proved feasible in this selected group and was well appreciated. Results showed a substantial drop in A1c at six-month follow-up, while emotional well-being was preserved.

The effectiveness of an extended (six-week) version of the programme was evaluated in a randomized, controlled trial. Participants, selected on long standing high HbA1c, report high levels of psychological distress and depressive symptoms, and self-efficacy was relatively low.[79] Results show that CBGT was successful in improving self-efficacy, diabetes-related distress and mood at three months follow-up, but not in improving glycaemic control.[80]

Weinger et al.[78] randomized type 1 diabetic patients to either a similar eight-week psychologist-led CBGT intervention, or cholesterol education classes to control for attention. The programme used cognitive restructuring and relaxation techniques to help participants achieve better glycaemic control. At six-month follow-up, adherence and HbA1c were improved in both groups. There were no differences in HbA1c between groups at post-test, although CBGT participants realized a modest improvement from pre- to post-test. Quality of life was improved in the experimental group only.

Overall, these short, structured interventions seem relatively effective in improving psychosocial functioning, even over the longer term. For interventions that are part of a more comprehensive educational programme, the relative benefit of coping skill training remains difficult to disaggregate. In adolescents, preventive intervening appears more effective when integrated with the start of intensive management.

7.7 Using New Technologies for Groups

The Internet provides health care professionals and patients with new opportunities to exchange not only information, but also support. Zrebiec and Jacobson[81] report on a World Wide Web-based educational and emotional resource for patients with diabetes. Over a period of 21 months, three professionally moderated discussion groups about nutrition, motivation and family issues were actively visited on the Internet. Visitors responding to a survey were mainly over 30 years old, both users and non-users of insulin, both recently diagnosed patients and those with long standing diabetes, and comprised a larger proportion of females than males. Nearly half of the users logged in more than three times, and 79 per cent rated participation as having a positive effect on their coping with diabetes.

A study by Barrera et al.[82] showed that the Internet is actually perceived by its users as an effective source of support. In a randomized trial, 160 novice Internet users with type 2 diabetes (53 per cent female; mean age 59.3 ± 9.4 years) were assigned to four Web-based conditions: diabetes information only, a personal self-management coach, or one of two interventions combining coaching and support. After three months, individuals in both support conditions reported significant increases in both diabetes-specific and general support.

7.8   Discussion and Future Directions

Reviewing the literature, it becomes clear that a group format may be applied in diabetes care either as a cost-effectiveness measure or to provide patients with the additional benefits that are inherent to group interventions, or both. Apart from instances involving long standing serious psychopathology, no evidence suggests the need to refrain from using groups for either reason.

To enhance psychosocial functioning and glycaemic control, interventions with a short, structured format seem to have more beneficial effects than groups relying on disclosure and sharing of experiences only. To achieve behavioural change, people need strategies and practice to translate new information into actual behaviours and to implement new behaviours in real life.

While this review shows many examples of interventions with beneficial effects, some limitations should be addressed.

Some populations that could greatly benefit from group interventions seem largely overlooked. For example, no accounts described group interventions for pregnant women, for preconception counselling in diabetes or painful neuropathy. Given that type 2 diabetes is now manifesting itself earlier in life, women may have an increasing need for support in this area.

As stated by many authors, there is still a dearth of well described interventions that are systematically evaluated through randomized trials with adequate sample sizes. Most studies lack the statistical power to draw unambiguous conclusions.

Another problem lies in the assessment of outcomes. When using generic instead of disease-specific measures, other factors (intra-individual, social, environmental) that may have an impact on, for example, quality of life, remain unappreciated. When assessing glycaemic control to evaluate the effectiveness of intervening at a psychosocial level, the processes mediating these effects are often overlooked. Psychosocial variables are addressed, which should result in behaviour changes, which in turn should influence glycaemic control. Often these processes remain a black box, and A1c is assessed directly after the intervention, before any resulting behavioural changes have actually had time to affect physiology.

Waiting-list control groups are frequently used in intervention studies. However, these provide no control for non-specific treatment factors (e.g. group support, expectation of success or placebo effects), and identifying the effective elements of treatment is difficult. Future studies should use control groups receiving equal amounts of health care contact to control for these factors.

The generalizability of results from research is constrained by low participation rates and high rates of participant drop-out. Results often apply only to highly motivated people, who are willing and able to engage in psychosocial interventions that require great commitment in terms of time and effort.

If psychologically orientated group interventions are to be integrated into routine clinical practice, there are a number of empirical issues that need to be addressed in the literature. First there is the rationale behind interventions, and a clear focus or theoretical process for an intervention. Reviewers of the literature have been consistent in commenting on the lack of theoretical rationale behind interventions, with one systematic review of psycho-educational interventions in adolescents establishing that just over half the studies in the field do not articulate how their intervention is supposed to work.[83] Furthermore, studies that did articulate their theoretical rationale had a substantially greater effect size. Theory is important as it enables professionals to be clear about what factor or variables they are targeting for change and how they are going to achieve change.

This links to the problems of the wider implementation of group programmes. If group programmes are to be integrated into routine practice, then non-psychological health professionals (medics, nurses, dietitians) will need to be recruited to deliver programmes. However, the literature continues to document the problems these professionals have with 1:1 consultations,[84] without adding the complexity and increased skill level required to effectively facilitate group programmes. This means researchers need to be clear about the training needs for individuals to deliver the programme, and the process by which quality assurance can be maintained. Finding methods that are objective assessments of process in groups is essential if programmes are to be effectively rolled out into routine practice. It is not unheard of for a health care professional to acquire a programme handbook, and even attend a brief training course. They then run a programme, with limited success, if any, and subsequently claim that the programme does not work.[85] However, experience tells us that there is little chance that the programme was delivered in the correct manner under this scenario, resulting in the lack of efficacy. Individuals need supporting in developing their general group facilitation skills and specific intervention skills and strategies. This is only achieved effectively through observation of programme delivery with supportive feedback.

If we resolve the problems with regard to the delivery of programmes there are still two methodological problems that studies need to address for health care to take on board the evidence. Many studies we have reported here, if not the majority, will have utilized a treatment as usual or wait list control group method. However, a group programme will normally result in a substantial increase in patient professional contact time. For example, a six-session programme of 90 min per session means the individual with diabetes now receives 9 hours of health care professional input into the management of their diabetes. In most countries this equates to more than 2 years of normal contact time with diabetes health care professionals. This is a substantial investment from the patient, and the professional. At the least, researchers need control for the professional per patient contact hours. For instance, in the above example, if we assume that the group has 12 people attending, and is facilitated by two professionals, we have 18 hours of professional time, to 12 patients, which equates to 1½ hours of professional input per patient. This is still more than many patients would get in a year of normal care. Therefore, researchers need to address this disparity, if groups are to be cost-effective approaches to be implemented in routine practice.

The last major methodological problem to address is the integration of clinical management with psycho-educational programmes. An group programme will only work if the individual is on the right treatment regimen. Changes in treatment regimen can affect glycaemic control and psychological well-being, by increasing flexibility of treatment, fitting treatment to a lifestyle, reducing medication-taking burden, reducing risks of hypoglycaemia etc. Therefore, it is essential that researchers do not see psycho-education programmes as acting in isolation from clinical care. The simplest way to address this is to have a run-in period before the intervention begins, where treatment regimen and diabetes skills (blood glucose monitoring) and knowledge are optimized and updated. This is relatively common practice in clinical trials of medication, but is an exception in psycho-educational research. Given the substantial effects that can be gained through an effective run-in period, this is a critical issue to address in the future.[86]

In conclusion, psychosocial interventions offered in a group format are a promising addition to diabetes care and education. There are many examples of well appreciated, effective, feasible interventions delivered by a wide range of professionals, not only behavioural therapists but also dietitians, diabetes educators and physicians. This confirms that, with proper training and experience, behavioural and cognitive techniques can be applied effectively by health care professionals outside the mental health specialties.

Future research should aim to translate interventions to other populations and settings, to develop new well described interventions on a theoretically sound basis, and to evaluate such interventions through well controlled, randomized study designs. The challenge for researchers and practitioners alike is to put this research into practice effectively.

References

1. Snoek FJ, Skinner TC. Psychological counseling in problematic diabetes: does it help? *Diabet Med* 2002; **19**: 265–273.
2. Rubin RR, Peyrot M. Psychosocial problems and interventions: a review of the literature. *Diabetes Care* 1992; **15**: 1640–1657.
3. Rubin RR, Peyrot M: Psychological issues and treatments for people with diabetes. *J Clin Psychol* 2001; **57**: 457–478.
4. Delamater AM, Jacobson AM, Anderson B, Cox D, Fisher L, Lustman P, Rubin R, Wysocki T. Psychosocial therapies in diabetes: report of the Psychosocial Therapies Working Group. *Diabetes Care* 2001; **24**: 1268–1292.
5. Lorenz RA, Bubb J, Davis D, Jacobson A, Jannasch K, Kramer J, Lipps J, Schlundt D. Changing behaviour: practical lessons from the Diabetes Control and Complications Trial. *Diabetes Care* 1996; **19**: 648–652.
6. Glasgow RE, Fisher EB, Anderson BJ, LaGreca A, MarreroD, Johnson SB, Rubin RR, Cox DJ. Behavioral science in diabetes: contributions and opportunities. *Diabetes Care* 1999; **22**: 832–843.

7. Skyler JS, Oddo C. Diabetes trends in the USA. *Diabetes Metab Res Rev* 2002; **18**: S21–S26.
8. Spira JL. Understanding and developing psychotherapy groups for medically ill patients. In Spira JL (ed), *Group Therapy for Medically Ill Patients*. New York, Guilford, 1997, pp 3–11.
9. Lorig KR, Sobel DS, Ritter PL, Laurent D, Hobbs M. Effect of a self-management program on patients with chronic disease. *Eff Clin Pract* 2001; **4**: 256–262.
10. Cox DJ, Irvine A, Gonder-Frederick L, Nowacek G, Butterfield J. Fear of hypoglycemia: quantification, validation, and utilization. *Diabetes Care* 1987; **10**: 617–621.
11. Vijan S, Stuart NS, Fitzgerald JT, Ronis DL, Hayward RA, Slater S, Hofer TP. Barriers to following dietary recommendations in Type 2 diabetes. *Diabet Med* 2005; **22**: 32–38.
12. DAFNE Study Group. Training in flexible, intensive insulin management to enable dietary freedom in people with Type 1 diabetes: Dose Adjustment for Normal Eating (DAFNE) randomized controlled trial. *Diabet Med* 2003; **20** (Suppl. 3): 4–5.
13. Murphy E, Kinmonth AL. No symptoms, no problem? Patients' understandings of non-insulin dependent diabetes. *Fam Pract* 1995; **12**: 184–192.
14. White CA. *Cognitive Behaviour Therapy for Chronic Medical Problems*. Chichester: Wiley, 2001.
15. Ellis SE, Speroff T, Dittus RS, Brown A, Pichert JW, Elasy TA. Diabetes patient education: a meta-analysis and meta-regression. *Patient Educ Couns* 2004; **52**: 97–105.
16. Steed L, Cooke D, Newman S. A systematic review of psychosocial outcomes following education, self-management and psychological interventions in diabetes mellitus. *Patient Educ Couns* 2003; **51**: 5–15.
17. Ismail K, Winkley K, Rabe-Hesketh S. Systematic review and meta-analysis of randomised controlled trials of psychological interventions to improve glycaemic control in patients with type 2 diabetes. *Lancet* 2004; **363**: 1589–1597.
18. Rachmani R, Levi Z, Slavachevski I, Avin M, Ravid M. Teaching patients to monitor their risk factors retards the progression of vascular complications in high-risk patients with Type 2 diabetes mellitus – a randomized prospective study. *Diabet Med* 2002; **19**: 385–392.
19. Trento M, Passera P, Borgo E, Tomalino M, Bajardi M, Cavallo F, Orta M. A 5-year randomized controlled study of learning, problem solving ability, and quality of life modifications in people with type 2 diabetes managed by group care. *Diabetes Care* 2004; **27**: 670–675.
20. Rickheim PL, Weaver TW, Flader JL, Kendall DM. Assessment of group versus individual diabetes education. A randomized study. *Diabetes Care* 2002; **25**: 269–274.
21. Anderson RJ, Freedland KE, Clouse RE, Lustman PJ. The prevalence of comorbid depression in adults with diabetes: a meta-analysis. *Diabetes Care* 2001; **24**: 1069–1078.
22. Dantzer C, Swendsen J, Maurice-Tison S, Salamon R. Anxiety and depression in juvenile diabetes: a critical review. *Clin Psychol Rev* 2003; **23**: 787–800.
23. De Groot M, Anderson R, Freedland KE, Clouse RE, Lustman PJ. Association of depression and diabetes complications: a meta-analysis. *Psychosom Med* 2001; **63**: 619–630.
24. Grigsby AB, Anderson RJ, Freedland KE, Clouse RE, Lustman PJ. Prevalence of anxiety in adults with diabetes. A systematic review. *J Pychosom Res* 2002; **53**: 1053–1060.
25. Anderson RJ, Grigsby AB, Freedland KE, de Groot M, McGill JB, Clouse RE, Lustman PJ. Anxiety and poor glycemic control: a meta-analytic review of the literature. *Int J Psychiatry Med* 2002; **32**: 235–247.
26. Surwit RS, van Tilburg MAL, Zucker N, McCaskill CC, Parekh P, Feinglos MN, Edwards CL, Williams P, Lane JD. Stress management improves long-term glycemic control in type 2 diabetes. *Diabetes Care* 2002; **25**: 30–34.
27. Aikens JE, Kiolbasa TA, Sobel R. Psychological predictors of glycemic change with relaxation training in non-insulin-dependent diabetes mellitus. *Psychother Psychosom* 1997; **66**: 302–306.

28. Stenström U, Göth A, Carlsson C, Andersson P. Stress management training as related to glycemic control and mood in adults with type 1 diabetes mellitus. *Diabetes Res Clin Pract* 2003; **60**: 147–152.

29. Yasar SA, Tulassay T, Madacsy L, Korner A, Szucs L, Nagy I, Szabo A, Miltenyi M. Sympathetic–adrenergic activity and acid–base regulation under acute physical stress in type I (insulin-dependent) diabetic children. *Horm Res* 1994; **42**: 110–115.

30. Riazi A, Pickup J, Bradley C. Daily stress and glycaemic control in Type 1 diabetes: individual differences in magnitude, direction, and timing of stress-reactivity. *Diabetes Res Clin Pract* 2004; **66**: 237–244.

31. Polonsky WH. *Diabetes Burnout: What To Do When You Can't Take It Anymore*. American Diabetes Association: Alexandra, 1999.

32. Rodin G, Olmsted MP, Rydall AC, Maharaj SI, Colton PA, Jones JM, Biancucci LA, Daneman D. Eating disorders in young women with type 1 diabetes mellitus. *J Psychosom Res* 2002; **53**: 943–949.

33. Alloway SC, Toth EL, McCargar LJ. Effectiveness of a group psychoeducation program for the treatment of subclinical disordered eating in women with type 1 diabetes. *Can J Diet Pract Res* 2001; **62**: 188–192.

34. Olmsted MP, Daneman D, Rydall AC, Lawson ML, Rodin G. The effects of psychoeducation on disturbed eating attitudes and behavior in young women with type 1 diabetes mellitus. *Int J Eat Disord* 2002; **32**: 230–239.

35. Kenardy J, Mensch M, Bowen K, Green B, Walton J. Group therapy for binge eating in type 2 diabetes: a randomized trial. *Diabet Med* 2002; **19**: 234–239.

36. Galatzer A, Amir S, Gil R, Karp M, Laron Z. Crisis intervention program in newly diagnosed diabetic children. *Diabetes Care* 1982; **5**: 414–419.

37. Spiess K, Sachs G, Pietschmann, Prager R. A program to reduce onset distress in unselected type I diabetic patients: effects on psychological variables and metabolic control. *Eur J Endocrinol* 1995; **132**: 580–586.

38. Snoek FJ, Pouwer F, Welch GW, Polonsky WH. Diabetes-related emotional distress in Dutch and U.S. diabetic patients: cross-cultural validity of the Problem Areas in Diabetes Scale. *Diabetes Care* 2000; **23**: 1305–1309.

39. Meltzer B, Egleston B. How patients with diabetes perceive their risk for major complications. *Eff Clin Pract* 2000; **3**: 7–15.

40. Frijling BD, Lobo CM, Keus IM, Jenks KM, Akkermans RP, Hulscher MEJL, Prins A, van der Wouden JC, Grol RPTM. Perceptions of cardiovascular risk among patients with hypertension or diabetes. *Patient Educ Couns* 2004; **1**: 47–53.

41. Oehler-Giarratana J. Meeting the psychosocial and rehabilitative needs of the visually impaired diabetic. *J Vis Impair Blindness* 1978; **72**: 358–361.

42. Caditz J. An education-support group program for visually impaired people with diabetes. *J Vis Impair Blindness* 1992; **96**: 81–83.

43. Bernbaum M, Albert SG, Brusca SR, Drimmer A, Duckro PN, Cohen JD, Trindade MC, Silverberg AB. A model clinical program for patients with diabetes and vision impairment. *Diabetes Educ* 1989; **15**: 325–330.

44. Zettler A, Duran G, Waadt S, Herschbach P, Strian F. Coping with fear of long-term complications in diabetes mellitus: a model clinical program. *Psychother Psychosom* 1995; **64**: 178–184.

45. Vileikyte L, Rubin R, Leventhal H. Psychological aspects of diabetic neuropathic foot complications: an overview. *Diabetes Metab Res Rev* 2004; **20** (Suppl. 1): S13–S18.

46. Ragnarson Tennvall G, Apelqvist J. Health-related quality of life in patients with diabetes mellitus and foot ulcers. *J Diabetes Complicat* 2000; **14**: 235–241.
Current foot ulcers and major amputations are associated with reduced health-related quality of life.

47. Benbow SJ, Cossins L, MacFarlane IA. Painful diabetic neuropathy. *Diabetic Med* 1999; **16**: 632–644.

48. Cox DJ, Gonder-Frederick LA, Julian DM, Clarke WL: *Blood Glucose Awareness Training III.* Charlottesville, VA: University of Virginia Health Sciences Center, 1995.

49. Cox DJ, Gonder-Frederick L, Polonsky W, Schlundt D, Julian D, Clarke W. A multicenter evaluation of Blood Gucose Awareness Training – II. *Diabetes Care* 1995; **18**: 523–528.

50. Cox DJ, Gonder-Frederick L, Polonsky W, Schlundt D, Kovatchev B, Clarke W. Blood Glucose Awareness training (BGAT-2): long-term benefits. *Diabetes Care* 2001; **24**: 637–642.

51. Kinsley BT, Weinger K, Bajaj M, Levy CJ, Simonson DC, Quigley M, Cox DJ, Jacobson AM. Blood Glucose Awareness Training and epinephrine responses to hypoglycemia during intensive treatment in type 1 diabetes. *Diabetes Care* 1999; **22**: 1022–1028.

52. Broers S, Le Cessie S, Van Vliet KP, Spinhoven Ph, van der Ven NCW, Radder JK. Blood Glucose Awareness Training in Dutch type 1 diabetes patients: short-term evaluation of individual and group training. *Diabet Med* 2002; **19**: 157–161.

53. Nurick MA, Johnson SB. Enhancing blood glucose awareness in adolescents and young adults with IDDM. *Diabetes Care* 1991; **14**: 1–7.

54. Kubiak T. *Entwicklung und erste empirische Ueberpruefung eines stationaeren Interventionskonzepts zur Behandlung von typ 1 Diabetikern mit Hypoglyakemieproblemen. [Development and First Empirical Evaluation of an Inpatient Intervention for the Treatment of Hypoglycaemia-Related Problems].* Frankfurt am Main: Lang, 2002 (in German).

55. Citrin WS, Furman SG, Girden E. Diabetes in adolescence: group assertiveness training and the traditional 'Rap' group. *Diabetes* 1983; **32** (Suppl. 1): 37A.

56. Follansbee DJ, La Greca AM, Citrin WS. Coping skills training for adolescents with diabetes. *Diabetes* 1983; **32** (Suppl. 1): 37A.

57. Smith KE, Schreiner B, Brouhard BH, Travis LB. Impact of a camp experience on choice of coping strategies by adolescents with insulin-dependent diabetes mellitus. *Diabetes Educ* 1991; **17**: 49–53.

58. Smith K, Schreiner B, Jackson C, Travis L. Teaching assertive communication skills to adolescents with diabetes: evaluation of a camp curriculum. *Diabetes Educ* 1993; **19**: 136–141.

59. Greco P, Sroff Pendley J, McDonell K, Reeves G. A peer group intervention for adolescents with type 1 diabetes and their best friends. *J Pediatr Psychol* 2001; **26**: 485–490.

60. Marrero DG, Myers GL, Golden MP, West D, Kershnar A, Lau N. Adjustment to misfortune: the use of a social support group for adolescent diabetics. *Pediatr Adolesc Endocrinol* 1982; **10**: 213–218.

61. Kaplan RM, Chadwick MW, Schimmel LE. Social learning intervention to promote metabolic control in type I diabetes mellitus: pilot experiment results. *Diabetes Care* 1985; **8**: 152–155.

62. Massouh SR, Steele TM, Alseth ER, Diekmann JM. The effect of social learning intervention on metabolic control of insulin-dependent diabetes mellitus in adolescents. *Diabetes Educ* 1989; **15**: 518–521.

63. Gross AM, Heimann L, Shapiro R, Schultz RM: Children with diabetes: social skills training with hemoglobin A1c levels. *Behav Mod* 1983; **7**: 151–164.

64. Boardway RH, Delamater AM, Tomakowsky J, Gutai JP: Stress management training for adolescents with diabetes. *J Pediatr Psychol* 1993; **18**: 29–45.

65. Grey M, Boland EA, Davidson M, Yu C, Sullivan-Bolyai S, Tamborlane WV. Short-term effects of coping skills training as adjunct to intensive therapy in adolescents. *Diabetes Care* 1998; **21**: 902–908.
66. Grey M, Boland EA, Davidson M, Li J, Tamborlane WV. Coping skills training for youth with diabetes mellitus has long-lasting effects on metabolic control and quality of life. *J Pediatr* 2000; **137**: 107–113.
67. Mendez FJ, Belendez M. Effects of a behavioral intervention on treatment adherence and stress management in adolescents with IDDM. *Diabetes Care* 1997; **20**: 1370–1375.
68. Viner RM, Christie D, Taylor V, Hey S. Motivational/solution-focused intervention improves HbA1c in adolescents with type 1 diabetes: a pilot study. *Diabet Med* 2003; **20**: 739–742.
69. Rabin C, Amir S, Nardi R, Ovadia B. Compliance and control: issues in group training for diabetics. *Health Soc Work* 1986; **11**: 141–151.
70. Rubin RR, Peyrot M, Saudek CD. Effect of diabetes education on self-care, metabolic control, and emotional well-being. *Diabetes Care* 1989; **12**: 673–679.
71. Rubin RR, Peyrot M, Saudek CD. The effect of a diabetes education program incorporating coping skills training on emotional well-being and diabetes self-efficacy. *Diabetes Educ* 1993; **19**: 210–214.
72. Bott U, Bott S, Hemmann D, Berger M. Evaluation of a holistic treatment and teaching programme for patients with type 1 diabetes who failed to achieve their therapeutic goals under intensified insulin therapy. *Diabet Med* 2000; **17**: 635–643.
73. Anderson RM, Funnell MM, Butler PM, Arnold MS, Fitzgerald JT, Feste CC. Patient empowerment: results of a randomized controlled trial. *Diabetes Care* 1995; **18**: 943–949.
74. Pibernik-Okanovic M, Prasek M, Poljicanin-Filipovic T, Pavlic-Renar I, Metelko Z. Effects of an empowerment-based psychosocial intervention on quality of life and metabolic control in type 2 diabetic patients. *Patient Educ Couns* 2004; **52**: 193–199.
75. Henry JL, Wilson PH, Bruce DG, Chisholm DJ, Rawling PJ. Cognitive–behavioural stress management for patients with non-insulin dependent diabetes mellitus. *Psychol Health Med* 1997; **2**: 109–118.
76. Schreurs KMG, Colland VT, Kuijer RG, De Ridder DTD, Van Elderen Th. Development, content and process evaluation of a short self-management intervention in patients with chronic diseases requiring self-care behaviours. *Patient Educ Couns* 2003; **51**: 13–141.
77. Snoek FJ, van der Ven NCW, Lubach CHC, Chatrou M, Ader HJ, Heine RJ, Jacobson AM. Effects of cognitive behavioral group training (CBGT) in adult patients with poorly controlled insulin-dependent (type 1) diabetes: a pilot study. *Patient Educ Couns* 2001; **45**: 143–148.
78. Weinger K, Schwartz E, Davis A, Rodriguez M, Simonson DC, Jacobson AM. Cognitive behavioral treatment in type 1 diabetes: a randomized control trial (Abstract). *Diabetes* 2002; **51** (Suppl. 2): A439.
79. Van der Ven NCW, Lubach CHC, Hogenelst MHE, Van Iperen A, Tromp-Wever AME, Vriend A, Van der Ploeg HM, Heine RJ, Snoek FJ. Cognitive Behavioural Group Training (CBGT) for patients with type 1 diabetes in persistent poor glycaemic control: who do we reach? *Patient Educ Couns* 2005; **56** (3): 313–322.
80. Van der Ven NCW, Hogenelst MHE, Tromp-Wever AME, Twisk JWR, Van der Ploeg HM, Heine RJ, Snoek FJ. Short term effects of Cognitive Behavioural Group Training (CBGT) in adult type 1 diabetes patients in prolonged poor glycaemic control. A randomised, controlled trial. *Diabet Med.* in press.
81. Zrebiec J, Jacobson AM. What attracts patients with diabetes to an internet support group? A 21-month longitudinal website study. *Diabet Med* 2001; **18**: 154–158.

82. Barrera M Jr, Glasgow RE, McKay HG, Boles SM, Feil EG. Do internet-based support interventions change perceptions of social support?: an experimental trial of approaches for supporting diabetes self-management. *Am J Commun Psychol* 2002; **30**: 637–654.

83. Hampson SE, Skinner TC, Hart J, Storey L, Gage H, Foxcroft D, Kimber A, Shaw K, Walker J. Effects of educational and psychosocial interventions for adolescents with diabetes mellitus: a systematic review. *Health Technol Assess* 2001; **5** (10): 1–79.

84. Parkin T, Skinner TC. Discrepancies between patient and professionals recall and perception of an outpatient consultation. *Diabet Med* 2003; **20**: 909–914.

85. Pill R, Rees ME, Stott NC, Rollnick SR. Can nurses learn to let go? Issues arising from an intervention designed to improve patients' involvement in their own care. *J Adv Nurs* 1999; **29**: 1492–1499.

86. De Vries JH, Snoek FJ, Kostense PJ, Heine RJ. Improved glycaemic control in type 1 diabetes pateints following participation per se in a clinical trial – mechanisms and implications. *Diabetes Metab Res Rev* 2003; **19**: 357–362.

8

Counselling and Psychotherapy in Diabetes Mellitus

Richard R. Rubin

8.1 Introduction

The importance of emotional issues in diabetes was first noted over 300 years ago in 1674 by Thomas Willis, the British physician who first recognized glycosuria in people with diabetes. Willis claimed that diabetes was caused by 'extreme sorrow'.[1] More recently, researchers have turned their attention from the emotional causes of diabetes to its emotional consequences. Over the past 25 years this research has greatly heightened our understanding of how common emotional problems are among patients with diabetes, and of how profoundly emotional problems affect diabetes outcomes. People who have diabetes frequently say they feel frustrated, fed up, overwhelmed or burned out by the demands of their disease. Polonsky and his associates found that approximately 60 per cent of respondents in their studies reported at least one serious diabetes-related distress, and that this distress was associated with less active self-care and higher A1c levels and rates of diabetes complications.[2] Frank psychological disorders, such as depression, are also a special problem for people with diabetes. Depression is more common in those who have diabetes. According to a recent study in a national representative sample of adults with diabetes, the 12-month incidence of major depressive disorder (MDD) was 9.3 per cent compared with a rate of 6.0 per cent in the general population.[3,4] Like diabetes-related distress, depression in patients with diabetes is associated with poorer regimen adherence,[5] and higher A1c levels,[6] complication rates,[5,7-9] and total health care costs.[5,10] Studies suggest that health care providers know how common emotional problems are among their patients with diabetes, and

Psychology in Diabetes Care   Edited by Frank J. Snoek and T. Chas Skinner
© 2005 John Wiley & Sons, Ltd.

that providers also recognize the impact of these problems on diabetes outcomes, but fewer providers feel able to treat these problems, and very few patients are referred for treatment.[11]

Very recently, other studies suggest that Willis might have been right after all; these studies found that people who are depressed are twice as likely to develop type 2 diabetes over a period of five years as people who are not depressed. This chapter will review what is known about the association between emotional problems (diabetes-related distress and frank psychopathology) and diabetes status and outcomes, as a foundation for describing and discussing counselling and psychotherapeutic approaches to improving emotional and metabolic outcomes in patients who have diabetes. We will start with a section on diabetes-related distress and proceed to a section on more serious emotional problems. We do not currently have a large body of evidence regarding the benefits of counselling or psychotherapy for diabetes patients, but we will discuss what we do know, as well as promising approaches that could prove beneficial.

8.2   Diabetes-Related Distress

The nature of diabetes-related distress

It is no wonder that diabetes distress is common. Living with diabetes presents countless challenges ranging from the mundane to the monumental, from finding time to check your blood glucose in the middle of a busy day to learning to live with the reality of a major diabetes complication.[12] Patients must deal with diabetes 24 hours a day, 365 days a year, or as a newly diagnosed 8-year-old patient pointed out to the author a few years ago, 366 days on Leap Year. Another patient noted that at least once every 15 minutes he stops briefly to check his 'diabetes temperature' pausing to consider whether he felt high or low, how long it had been since he had eaten, when he had last taken insulin, what he would be doing in the next hour or two and whether he should check his blood glucose level. This kind of attention to the treatment regimen is the key to optimizing outcomes. Since this regimen involves essentially everything the person does, for most people good diabetes care involves significant changes in lifestyle. We ask all of our patients to eat carefully, exercise regularly and monitor their blood glucose levels as recommended, and we ask many of them to take medication to help them keep their glucose, blood pressure and cholesterol levels as close to normal as possible. A recent study of people with type 2 diabetes found that half of a sample took at least seven different medications every day,[13] reminding us that the diabetes self-care regimen is complex, generally unpleasant and unremitting, involving many impositions and restrictions. Few people would choose to eat as carefully and stay as active as people with diabetes are supposed to, and no one would choose to follow the regimen of medication taking, blood glucose monitoring and medical follow-up recommended for most people with diabetes. Some advances in diabetes treatment reduce the burden of diabetes self-care, but others lead to recommendations for more intensive and demanding self-care.

Patients often find meeting these demands especially challenging because their efforts are not guaranteed to produce positive results. Hard work increases the chances for good outcomes, but it does not guarantee them; patients frequently report daily fluctuations in blood glucose levels when following the same regimen every day.

High and low blood sugars themselves add to the stress of living with diabetes. Hyperglycaemia is associated with reduced energy levels[14] and poorer cognitive functioning,[15,16] contributing significantly to higher levels of emotional distress and poorer quality of life.[6,16–19] Hypoglycaemia is also associated with distress. The acute effects of hypoglycaemia range from transient discomfort, to embarrassment when neuroglycopenia affects behaviour, to emergencies when hypoglycaemia is profound or it occurs when a person is driving. Some people greatly fear hypoglycaemia,[20] and a few purposefully keep their blood glucose levels high enough to make low glucose levels highly unlikely, but dramatically increase the risk of diabetes complications.[21]

Fear of taking insulin is another common source of diabetes-related distress. A recent large-scale international survey of adults with diabetes and clinicians from 13 countries in Asia, Australia, Europe and North America called the Diabetes Attitudes, Wishes, and Needs (DAWN) study found that almost half (48 per cent) of all patients not yet taking insulin believed that initiating insulin therapy meant they had failed to follow treatment recommendations, while only 23 per cent believed taking insulin would help them control their diabetes.[22] Patients often have other serious worries about starting insulin, including the fear that it means diabetes is worsening, that life will be more complicated or that insulin will cause diabetes complications.[23,24]

Diabetes is a family disease because it affects everyone who loves, lives with or cares for a person who has diabetes, and how all these people respond affects how the person with diabetes feels, and how that person takes care of his or her diabetes. Patients who feel unsupported or hassled say it is a major source of distress. Feeling unsupported or hassled by family and friends is yet another source of distress. Some patients feel that family and friends tempt them to ignore their diabetes or do not support their efforts to manage the disease (e.g. 'Eat a little cake; a bite won't hurt you' or 'Why do we always have to wait for dinner until after you test your blood?'). Others feel their family (and friends) go to the opposite extreme, monitoring and criticizing every action that could affect blood glucose levels (e.g. 'You know that cookie is not on your diet; are you trying to kill yourself?' or 'You haven't walked in weeks. You'll never control your diabetes that way'). Some patients report that their family and friends fluctuate between providing too little support and harassing them. Both lack of support and criticism add stress to the life of a person who has diabetes, often generating feelings of isolation, frustration, anger and guilt. This distress is a problem in its own right, and these feelings also can compromise self-care, physical well-being and the quality of a person's most important relationships.

Treating diabetes-related distress: psycho-educational interventions

The key to effectively treating diabetes-related distress is enhancing the patients coping skills. Approaches focus on helping patients either avoid stressful situations or helping patients manage stressful situations they cannot avoid, with many interventions focusing on both.

A wide range of interventions, including therapy groups, self-help groups support groups and diabetes camps for children have been employed to promote more effective coping in children and adults with diabetes. Most studies in children and adolescents have been designed to help participants cope more effectively with social situations that put regimen adherence at risk, using peer modelling and role play in group settings. These studies reported benefits such as greater emotional well-being,[25,26] enhanced coping skills,[27,28] better regimen adherence[27,29,30] and improved glycaemic control.[27,29,31] Grey and her colleagues reported that adolescents who practiced intensive diabetes management and received coping skill training had lower A1c levels, had more confidence in their ability to manage their diabetes, and reported less impact of diabetes on their quality of life than adolescents who practiced intensive management but did not receive coping skill training.[32,33] Wysocki and colleagues reported mixed results for the families of adolescents who participated in a trial of behavioural family systems therapy (BFST). Participants in this group had better parent–adolescent relationships, but no improvement in adjustment to diabetes or glycaemic control, compared with those receiving standard treatment.[34]

Diabetes camps usually include formal or informal interventions to enhance the coping skills of young campers. Reported benefits of attending diabetes camp include an enhanced sense of diabetes self-efficacy.[35,36] Unfortunately, most reports are restricted to interventions for children and adolescents, and few studies included a control group or follow-up measures to assess long term benefits, so the evidence for specific approaches is not as strong as we would like. The two camp studies that incorporated control groups found no differences in psychosocial outcomes between campers and non-campers.[37,38]

In contrast, Marrero and colleagues[39] found that adolescents who participated in a series of sessions designed to improve diabetes-related coping skills were less depressed, and also tended to have higher self-esteem and more often used emotion-based coping skills, when compared with a control group. In another controlled trial, Anderson and her colleagues[40] provided separate group sessions for adolescents and their parents as a supplement to regular diabetes clinic visits. The goal of the adolescent sessions was to increase skill in using SMBG data for regimen adjustments. The goal of the parent sessions was to develop strategies for negotiating appropriate levels of parental involvement in the adolescent's diabetes care. Eighteen months after completion of the 12-session group intervention, adolescents in the treatment group had significantly lower A1c levels and reported significantly more use of SMBG data for selected regimen adjustments than adolescents in the control group.

Group psychosocial interventions (see Chapter 7) have also been employed with adults who have diabetes. These groups specifically address coping difficulties rather than frank psychopathology; reported benefits of these studies, which also often lack control groups, adequate statistical power or follow-up assessments, include increases in emotional well-being,[41–47] coping skills,[45–47] regimen adherence,[45] and glycaemic control.[43] One controlled trial in this area found that a group-based counselling programme focussed on coping with diabetes resulted in reduced diabetes-related distress, improved coping and better glycaemic control.[41] The other controlled study in this area found an increase in psychological well-being and social functioning, but these improvements did not differ significantly from those achieved by a lecture-only control group, and neither group improved in glycaemic control.[47]

In some settings, coping skill training is incorporated into broader programmes of self-management education. In fact, the American Diabetes Association (ADA) has stated that psychosocial issues must be addressed by all diabetes education programmes it certifies.[48] The Johns Hopkins University Diabetes Center offers a diabetes self-management education programme that incorporates diabetes-specific coping skills training (CST) designed to help patients overcome barriers to the successful application of new knowledge and skills. This intervention is designed to improve patients' emotional well-being, diabetes self-care and long term blood glucose control. The CST approach used in this programme is a psycho-educational group intervention that addresses attitudes and behaviours that underlie individual patterns of self-care; this approach has been described in detail elsewhere.[49–51] In a group setting, individuals begin the process by identifying their own personal regimen barriers or 'sticking points'. Patients are encouraged to identify sticking points as specifically as possible; the more specifically the sticking point is defined, the easier it is to resolve. Once a personal issue has been identified, patients help each other develop strategies for dealing with these issues, focusing on strategies that have been successful in the past. A key goal of this process is to help patients recognize that certain thoughts or attitudes trigger distress and non-constructive behaviour, while other thoughts and attitudes trigger a process that leads to better outcomes.[52] Patients learn that the ability to focus on thoughts that lead to desired outcomes is a skill that can be developed through persistent practice. A final element of the coping skill training intervention is relapse prevention,[53] designed to help patients develop techniques for coping with the inevitable occasions when motivation wanes and self-care and emotional well-being slip. A case example of the coping skill training intervention is described in

Table 8.1   Coping skill training example

First Session (90 minutes)

- *Identify specific regiment problem:* 'grazing' (continuous nibbling) after dinner
- *Identify 'trigger' thoughts for failure:* 'I've already blown my diet (after the first nibble) so it makes no difference what I do now
- *Identify 'trigger' thoughts for success (personal or generated by the group):* 'I've done pretty well with my diet all day. If I stop after nibble I can still feel good about myself and I won't be up all night going to the toilet'
- *Practice 'trigger' thoughts for success:* based on a common problem, group participants visualize the problem situation and rehearse solutions

Between Sessions

- *Implement coping skills:* at home, implement approaches learned in first session
- *Identify successful and less-than-successful outcomes:* 'I grazed less than usual, but I did not stop altogether'

Second Session (60 minutes)

- *Refine coping approaches:* add coping tactics, e.g. preparing acceptable snack and then not re-entering kitchen for the rest of the evening, identifying non-food treats (music, social contacts) and incorporate them into evening routine
- *Develop relapse prevention techniques:* 'contracts for change' are completed by all participants. Contracts include cognitive elements ('Remember, everybody slips; your goal is to keep a lapse from becoming a collapse') and behaviour ('When you lapse, use your support network – family, friends, medical staff and especially other group members'). Group participants are provided with a list of members' phone numbers and encouraged to call when in need of support

Table 8.1. The first coping skill training session is held the morning of the second day of the group education programme, and the second session is held on the afternoon of the fourth day.

The benefits of this psycho-educational programme are wide ranging and robust, as demonstrated in a series of studies.[51,54–58] Patients who participated in the education programme reported higher levels of emotional well-being (self-esteem, diabetes self-efficacy, depression and anxiety) and self-care behaviour (SMBG frequency, medication adherence and adjustment, diet and exercise) six and 12 months after completing the intervention than they had when they entered the programme, and their A1c levels were lower, as well. Because the overall educational programme has multiple components, it is not possible to determine which aspects of the intervention, alone or in combination, were responsible for the positive outcomes associated with participation. However, the coping skill training component, which took up two of the 37 hours patients spent in the programme, could have helped persons to deal with their problems in living with diabetes. It has been demonstrated that effective coping is associated with better self-management and glycaemic control and can reduce the deleterious effects of stress.[59–60]

In the Hopkins programme the additional cost of the CST component was about $35 per patient. The most difficult obstacle to establishing coping skill training programmes within diabetes educational interventions may be identifying a professional who is sufficiently experienced in diabetes-specific coping skill training. If such a professional is not available, two approaches should be considered: identifying a mental health professional who is interested in developing diabetes-specific expertise, or enhancing the counselling skills of providers who are not mental health professionals.

Treating diabetes-related distress: clinical interventions

Clinicians can incorporate elements of the CST approach into their regular interactions with patients. Doing this effectively enhances patients' coping skills and increases the likelihood of associated beneficial outcomes. Providers can do this by keeping in mind the CST techniques that make success more likely.

Ask good questions

We can begin helping patients cope better with diabetes by asking questions that help them identify sources of their own diabetes-related distress. Start with questions such as these: 'How are things going with your diabetes?', 'What concerns you most about your diabetes?' and 'What is the hardest thing for you right now about living with diabetes?'. To be most useful, the patients' responses should be very specific. To illustrate the benefits of focussing on a very specific 'sticking point', we offer the following example. A man sought treatment from the author, stating he was a 'bad diabetic' who did 'nothing right'. A few questions uncovered the man's specific sticking point: no matter what he tried, he could not stop snacking between dinner and bedtime. As a result, the man was up many times each night to urinate (a result of hyperglycaemia), and he dragged himself through the next day exhausted, guilty and discouraged.

Identifying a specific sticking point is often a source of relief for patient and provider alike, because it clarifies the fact the patient is not doing as badly as he believed he was, and because it provides a focussed target for intervention. Patients often describe their diabetes coping challenges in broad terms; they may say that everything bothers them, or they may focus to a degree, and say their major difficulty is their diet. With encouragement (e.g. suggesting that the patient describe the problem clearly enough for you to take a picture or make a video of it) almost every person can identify more specific sticking points.

Focus on successes

A sticking point is by definition a place where a person often gets stuck, but most people can recall instances when the outcome was better than it usually is. So one of the most important and useful questions to ask is 'How come it worked better that time?'. This approach helped with the evening snacker I just described. This man had occasionally avoided excess snacking even before he sought treatment for his problem. As we talked about these rare successes the patient realized that he managed to control his eating when he thought about his young grandson, when he would say to himself, 'I want to be alive 15 years from now to see that boy walk across the stage and get his high school diploma'. That seemed to work.

Helping patients figure out what makes things work better on certain occasions helps them improve coping skills and self-care, and it helps in the most effective possible way, by focussing on successes rather than on failures.

Support problem-solving skills

When a person has diabetes, achieving good physical and emotional health requires good problem-solving skills. Many patients learn to develop such skills. A teenager who had only a few days earlier begun using an insulin pump was planning to go out to dinner with his father. The meal was a special occasion, and the young man had talked his father into letting him eat anything he wanted. Unfortunately, the boy's pre-dinner blood glucose level was 350 mg/dl. Despite his trepidation, the father agreed to stick with the agreement on the condition that the young man think really hard about how much insulin he needed to take to cover the meal and that he test his blood 2 hours and 4 hours after dinner. Even after a big dinner, the results of these tests were 220 mg/dl and 150 mg/dl. The boy explained his success: 'I calculated how much carbohydrate was in each thing I ate, and I used the formula I was taught to figure the amount of insulin I needed. I really wanted that food, and I really didn't want to feel sick later, so I worked hard to get the insulin right'.

Involve the family

As noted earlier, diabetes is a family disease: the demands of diabetes and its management affect everyone who loves, lives with or cares for a person who has diabetes. Moreover, the behaviour of those who are close to them affects the way people take care of their diabetes. The most appropriate help for a patient with support problems depends on the specific situation. If family members' lack of support or over-involvement stems from a lack of knowledge or understanding about diabetes and diabetes care, attending diabetes education classes or reading books or magazines that discuss these issues might be helpful. Meeting with the person who has diabetes and his or her family might also facilitate more constructive interaction and communication. If the patient or family members do not choose to meet in this setting, asking the person with diabetes some basic questions may help. The patient should be asked to offer examples of ways family and friends make it easier to manage diabetes, examples of ways they make it harder to manage diabetes and specific, realistic changes others could make that would help the person feel more supported or less harassed. Counselling the patient in ways to effectively communicate a desire for change will facilitate the process. Finally, some people with diabetes benefit from participating in diabetes support groups organized by local hospitals.

Help build emotional strength

Coping effectively with diabetes requires emotional strength as well as problem-solving skills. The fundamental elements of this emotional strength are love, faith and humour. Clinicians can foster these qualities in themselves and their patients. It is said that love conquers all, and when it comes to coping with the stress of life with diabetes this may well be true. Love gives us confidence, and it just plain feels wonderful. Help patients recognize the power of this positive emotion, so the hassles and aggravations of daily life with diabetes do not prevent patients and their families from enjoying, appreciating and loving each other.

Optimism is another antidote to diabetes distress. Help patients and their families draw personal sources of hope and optimism. Think about the fortitude and creativity many patients display. Forty years ago, a 13-year-old became the first person in her family to be diagnosed with diabetes. When the girl asked her mother what having diabetes would mean for them, her mother responded 'It means we will learn to eat better than we have ever eaten before, we will all be healthier than we ever were before, and we will all learn to love each other more than we ever did before'.

The author spoke with a 54-year-old man several months after the patient was diagnosed with diabetes. After noting his difficulties adjusting to some aspects of his new regimen, he quickly added 'It's not all bad. I've started walking in the evenings, and that has been just great. My wife and I head out after dinner at least 3 nights a week. We walk and talk. We've been married 33 years, and I don't think we've ever felt closer. And that's not all, we've each lost a few pounds and we feel good about that'.

Humour is also a powerful source of emotional strength. Along with faith, it's the closest thing to magic in the world. How often has someone said 'I don't know how I would have made it if it hadn't been for my sense of humour?'. Humour helps keep things in perspective; it protects people from feeling overwhelmed. If clinicians can help patients and their families apply humour to their lives with diabetes, they will be providing them with a real service.

The essence of humour is taking a bad situation and exaggerating its awfulness to the point it is so ridiculous it becomes funny. Fortunately or unfortunately, life with diabetes presents us with plenty of material for humour. Ask patients if anything funny has ever happened to them related to their diabetes. That question brought the following response from one woman I treated. She had awakened in the middle of the night in the throes of a hypoglycaemic reaction. Her usual antidotes (graham crackers and juice) were not by her bed, and she was too shaky to make it down to the kitchen herself, so she awakened her husband. He dragged himself out of bed and staggered groggily down the stairs. As the minutes ticked by the woman lay in bed waiting and shaking from her reaction. Finally, she started to crawl out of bed to get the food she needed (and to find out what had happened to her husband), when he came staggering back up the stairs, still half asleep–and empty handed! 'Where is my food?' the woman cried. 'Oh no! I ate it myself', he chagrined husband responded. Needless to say, his second trip to the kitchen for food was quicker than the first had been. In a few minutes the woman's blood glucose level was headed back to normal. At that point they shared a good laugh about how ridiculous the situation had been and quickly went peacefully and happily back to sleep.

Identifying and discussing any loving, hopeful or humorous diabetes-related experiences can help patients cope better with their disease. These experiences are rare for most people, but recognizing they exist at all may have a powerful salutary effect, relieving distress in the moment, and enhancing motivation for diabetes care in the long run.

8.3   Psychopathology

Patients with diabetes experience disproportionately high rates of psychological disorders, as do patients suffering from other serious chronic medical conditions. Depression and anxiety disorders are the most common diagnoses among people with diabetes, and these conditions occur more often in these patients than in the general population.[3,4,61,62] Clinically diagnosable eating disorders also appear to be more prevalent among people with diabetes than in the general population; this association is especially strong in young women.[63–66] Whether or not eating disorders are more common among patients with diabetes, these disorders clearly present special problems for these patients because of their association with an increased risk for diabetes complications.[67] Depression, anxiety and eating disorders can all be treated effectively, but they all tend to recur and they may require repeated treatment. Below we provide a detailed discussion of these disorders among people who have diabetes, and review the validated psychological treatments for each disorder. We begin with the most studied disorder, depression.

Depression screening

Patients at elevated risk for depression can be identified through the medical history and clinical presentation, and by asking depression-specific questions or through use of depression screening tools. Patients with a history of depression, anxiety disorder, mental health treatment, substance abuse or smoking are at heightened risk for depression, as are women, and those with a family history of depression or mental health treatment. Women are more likely to be depressed than men are. Patients who have multiple complications are more likely to be depressed, especially when these complications include neuropathy, impotence or cardiovascular disease.[7,68]

Patients who complain of chronic pain or symptoms out of proportion to their apparent physical basis, patients who have multiple vague complaints and patients who appear unable to manage their diabetes and who make heavy use of health care services are also at elevated risk for depression.

According to the DSM-IV,[69] nine symptoms are characteristic of depression (see Table 8.2). Depressed mood and loss of interest and pleasure are considered the

Table 8.2 Symptoms of clinical depression

1. Depressed mood (feeling sad or empty) most of the day, nearly every day
2. Significant weight loss when not dieting, or weight gain (e.g. a change of more than 5% of body weight in a month), or decrease or increase in appetite nearly every day
3. Trouble sleeping or sleeping too much nearly every day
4. Feeling really agitated or really sluggish physically nearly every day
5. Fatigue or loss of energy nearly every day
6. Markedly diminished interest or pleasure in all, or almost all, activities most of day, nearly every day
7. Feeling worthless or excessively or inappropriately guilty nearly every day
8. Diminished ability to think or concentrate, on indecisiveness, nearly every day
9. Recurrent thoughts of death (not just fear of dying), recurrent thoughts of suicide, or a suicide attempt or a specific plan to commit suicide

cardinal symptoms, and at least one must be present for a diagnosis of depression. Clinicians should be aware that people can be depressed and suffer the consequences of depression without reporting depressed mood. Four of the secondary symptoms are physical – change in sleep, change in appetite/weight, low energy/fatigue and psychomotor agitation or retardation. The remaining three secondary symptoms are cognitive or mental: poor concentration, low self-esteem/guilt and recurrent thoughts of death or suicide. For a diagnosis of major depressive disorder (MDD), the most serious and most researched form of depression, *five or more* of these nine symptoms must be present (including *one or both* cardinal symptoms) nearly every day for at least 2 weeks and must cause significant distress or dysfunction. Other common depression-related diagnoses in patients with diabetes include dysthymic disorder (depressed mood + at least two other DSM-IV depression symptoms, more days than not, without major depressive episode over two-year period) and adjustment disorder with depressed mood (depressed mood, tearfulness or feelings of hopelessness associated with a specific stressor, e.g. being diagnosed with diabetes or developing a complication). Studies that classified patients by level of likely depression have found that even mild depression is associated with poorer diabetes outcomes.[7,70]

Some physical symptoms of depression are the same as symptoms of hyperglycaemia or other diabetes symptoms, and this can present problems for the general clinician attempting to identify patients with diabetes who may be depressed. One study found that non-psychiatric physicians could identify more than 90 per cent of the depression cases in a population of patients, many in poor control and with advanced complications, using a standard psychiatric interview, even when symptoms attributable to diabetes were disallowed.[71] This was accomplished by focussing on the primary symptoms of depression and the secondary cognitive and mental symptoms. On the other hand, another study suggests that physical symptoms of diabetes can actually help identify depressed patients. In this study, patients who reported more physical diabetes symptoms, including fatigue, blurred vision, thirst, parathesias and polyuria, were also more likely to be depressed – even after controlling for diabetes severity, medical co-morbidity and HbA1c.[70] The latter finding suggests that clinicians should strongly consider screening for depression in diabetic patients who present with symptoms of hyperglycaemia or other diabetes symptoms that seem out of proportion with clinical indicators of metabolic control.

The clinician can identify patients likely to be depressed by asking two questions about mood and anhedonia (the DSM-IV cardinal diagnostic criteria): 'During the past 2 weeks, have you felt depressed, tearful or hopeless?' and 'During the past 2 weeks, have you felt little interest or pleasure in doing things you used to enjoy?'. Positive responses to one or both questions should trigger questions about the remaining seven DSM-IV symptoms, verifying the severity, frequency and duration of any symptoms that are present. Clinicians can also choose from a variety of validated self-report questionnaires for depression screening. These questionnaires take a patient less than 5 minutes to complete, and scoring takes less than 2 minutes, so results are available to discuss at the same visit. The Patient Health Questionnaire – 9 (PHQ-9),[72] which has questions that match the DSM-IV diagnostic criteria for depression, was recently introduced and is now being widely used. Other depression screeners, including the Beck Depression Inventory (BDI),[73] and the Center for Epidemiologic Studies Depression Scale (CES-D),[74] have established scores indicating likely mild, moderate and severe depression. The WHO-5 Well Being Index may also be useful for identifying depression, especially in elderly patients.[75–77]

Depression treatment

Investigators at Washington University School of Medicine (St. Louis, MO) conducted three separate, short term (8–10 weeks), controlled clinical trials to examine the efficacy of tricyclic antidepressants (nortriptyline),[78] selective serotonin reuptake inhibitors (fluoxetine)[79] and psychotherapy (cognitive behaviour therapy)[80] for major depression in people with diabetes. The results suggest that treatments that work in the general population work for people with diabetes as well. In each of the three studies conducted at Washington University, reduction in the severity of depression symptoms was significantly greater with the active compared to the control treatment, and remission of depression was uniformly higher in the treated group compared with the control group (nortriptyline, 57 versus 35 per cent; fluoxetine, 62 versus 31 per cent; cognitive therapy, 85 versus 27 per cent).

In addition, each study found that improvements in depression symptoms had beneficial effects on glucose regulation as measured by glycosylated hemoglobin (HbA1c) levels. While these findings are encouraging and the studies were well controlled, the number of patients studied was small. More recent randomized trials with larger numbers of patients who had much better blood glucose control produced different results: depression treatment improved depression but changes in addition to glucose control did not differ from those of a group not receiving the depression treatment.[81,82]

In the Washington University cognitive therapy study,[80] the control group received an educational intervention aimed at tighter glycaemic control combined with supportive counselling by a nurse or other diabetes educator. This approach led to remission of depression in only 27 per cent of cases, a rate only one-third as effective as the active treatment (cognitive behaviour therapy) and not generally different from the placebo response rate observed in psychiatric trials. This study strongly suggests that effective relief from depression requires depression-specific psychotherapeutic management.

The researchers also found that hyperglycaemia and the presence of diabetes complications predicted diminished response to depression treatment in both the nortriptyline and cognitive therapy trials.[78,80] Pretreatment HbA1c level was significantly lower in patients who responded to depression treatment compared with those who did not ($p < 0.05$ for each comparison). Taken together, these findings suggest that those in better glycaemic control respond better to depression treatment and that those who respond better to depression treatment improve their glycaemic control. This makes clear the need for a comprehensive management approach that simultaneously focuses on improved glycaemic control and relief of depression symptoms.

Decisions regarding depression treatment should be informed by the fact that depression in diabetes is a chronic condition, with relapse rates of approximately 80 per cent over five-year intervals.[83] Relapse following successful treatment is the norm, and few subjects remain asymptomatic for more than a year. Cognitive–behavioural therapy benefits were sustained at six months, but we do not know the ultimate duration of this effect. The chronicity of depression is increasingly recognized, and the benefits of maintenance treatment (i.e. continuing patients on antidepressant medications beyond the point of depression remission) has been established in psychiatric samples. Patrick Lustman described a significant advantage of maintenance medication therapy for depression in diabetes. At 12-month follow-up, patients receiving maintenance treatment were at least 20 per cent less likely to suffer a relapse into depression than a group of patients whose depression medication was discontinued when their symptoms remitted.[84] These findings indicate the benefits of chronic depression treatment for patients with diabetes.[82]

Anxiety disorder prevalence and screening

Prevalence studies using structured diagnostic interviews have found that people with diabetes have elevated rates of generalized anxiety disorder and simple phobia compared with the general population.[85–87] Other research[88] suggests that people who have diabetes may suffer from high anxiety levels as frequently as they do high depression symptom levels, and at much higher rates than the general population. The presence of more complications of diabetes also was significantly associated with high levels of anxiety, as it is with elevated symptoms of depression.

Anxiety disorders, like depression, often are undiagnosed and untreated in patients with diabetes; the under-diagnosis may be a result of mistaking common physical symptoms of anxiety for those of hypoglycaemia and misidentifying an anxiety disorder as poor adjustment to diabetes.

There are few studies of the effects of anxiety on metabolic control in people with diabetes, but it appears that severe anxiety, like depression, may interfere with diabetes self-care, and it may thus affect metabolic control indirectly. One study showed that an anxious coping style was associated with increased stress, reduced regimen adherence and poorer glycaemic control.[60] The results of efforts to study the direct psychophysiologic effects of anxiety (often conceived of as stress) on glycaemia in people with diabetes have been inconsistent; some studies reporting hyperglycaemic responses to stress, while others found no such response.[60]

Anxiety disorder treatment

Biofeedback-assisted relaxation training (BART) has been shown to improve glucose tolerance and reduced long term hyperglycaemia in people with type 2 diabetes,[31] but the effectiveness of BART for those with type 1 diabetes is less clear cut, although some studies have reported positive findings.[89] Little research has been done on the effectiveness of most stress management or psychotherapeutic interventions in patients with diabetes suffering from high levels of anxiety, though Zettler *et al.* found that in a small group of patients behaviourally oriented group therapy improved coping with fear of diabetes-related complications.[90] Other treatments validated in the general population should also be considered.

Psychopharmacological agents can be effective in the treatment of anxiety disorders in the general population, but there is little information on the use of these medications in patients who have diabetes. In one study, treatment with a benzodiazepine (fludiazepam) in a small group of patients with type 2 diabetes resulted in decreased anxiety ratings as well as an improvement in lipoproteins.[91] Another study reported improved glycaemic control in patients treated with alprazolam, although not all patients had a diagnosed anxiety disorder.[92] Benzodiazepines can be highly addictive, so they should be used cautiously. Using SSRIs to treat anxiety disorders is increasingly popular; a benzodiazepine may be prescribed in combination with the SSRI, and the benzodiazepine may be discontinued when a therapeutic level of the SSRI has been reached.

Eating disorder prevalence and screening

The true prevalence of eating disorders among people with diabetes is unknown, in part because in patients with diabetes it is hard to distinguish between a focus on food and the body, which is a necessary part of life with diabetes, and the abnormal concerns and behaviour that are used to diagnose eating disorder.[93] In the eating disordered behaviours people with type I diabetes share with the general population of patients with eating disorders, those with type 1 diabetes often engage in a variant unique to those taking insulin. Recent research suggests that between one-third and one-half of all young women with type 1 diabetes engage in *insulin purging*, deliberately taking less insulin than they need for good glycaemic control, in order to control their weight.[67] When patients engage in this behaviour, blood glucose levels remain high, fat storage is inhibited, and excess glucose passes from the blood, and is then excreted in the urine. Many eating disordered persons with type 1 diabetes say that insulin purging is easier and less unpleasant than vomiting. Binge eating is relatively common in people with type 2 diabetes, with estimates of disordered eating in this population ranging from five to 25 per cent.[94–97]

Clinical eating disorders, and even sub-clinical eating disordered behaviour, are associated with poor glycaemic control,[94–100] and higher rates of diabetes complications[101] and mortality.[102] Several researchers have found that insulin manipulation *per se* is associated with poor metabolic control,[103] and an increased risk for diabetic complications.[67,104,105] Persons with eating disorders are also less likely to follow recommendations regarding non-diet aspects of the diabetes regimen,[99,106] reflecting the underlying psychological pathology.

Eating disorder treatment

Treating eating disorders is a major challenge whether or not the patient has diabetes, because patients with eating disorders often resist acknowledging the problem. A high percentage of persons with recurrent diabetic ketoacidosis (RDKA), especially young women, are likely to have eating disorders, particularly insulin purging.[107] It is important that this behaviour be probed in addition to conventional symptoms. Eating disorders in diabetes may be responsive to psychotherapy, but the number of published intervention studies is small, and several of these lack methodological rigour. There is some evidence that CBT may be effective in treating individuals with mild to moderate eating disorders in the early stages.[108] Psychotherapeutic interventions should address the complex of underlying issues that often cause and sustain eating disordered behaviour–depression, diminished self-esteem and excessive dependence as well as risk-taking behaviour such as substance abuse and sexual acting out.[93] Established eating disorders are very difficult to treat on an outpatient basis; it is best to liaise with or refer patients to centres specialized in treating eating disorders.

Given how difficult it is to treat established eating disorders, clinicians should engage in primary prevention efforts for these disorders, especially in young female patients who have diabetes. These strategies include addressing the drive for thinness and associated body dissatisfaction, de-emphasizing dieting, counselling patients about the need to express negative feelings about diabetes self-management, addressing metabolic reactivity during adolescence, helping the patient with conflict over normal developmental struggles and working with the family.[109] Mental health professionals can help general clinicians implement these primary prevention strategies.

Some antidepressants in the SSRI class (including fluoxetine, paroxetine and sertraline) and closely related agents such as venlafaxine have been used to treat compulsive behaviour, including eating disordered behaviour, in the general population. On this basis, these medications should be considered when treating these problems in patients with diabetes.

Other psychological disorders

A variety of other psychological disorders create special problems for patients with diabetes.[110] Schizophrenia and substance abuse can compromise the patient's ability to manage diabetes. Alcoholism can have unanticipated consequences because alcohol interferes with the ability of the liver to store and release glucose in service of glucose homeostasis.[111] Obsessive compulsive disorder can lead patients to monitor blood glucose incessantly with no enhancement in glucose control. Phobic disorders can create obstacles to taking insulin and finger sticks for blood glucose monitoring. However, other than alcoholism, these disorders are not common. Nevertheless, when treating patients with these disorders, clinicians should be aware of the ways these disorders affect diabetes self-management and consequent health outcomes.

8.4 Practice Implications

In this chapter I have reviewed counselling and psychotherapeutic interventions for patients with diabetes who are having difficulties coping with the day-to-day demands of life with diabetes, and for patients who suffer from frank psychopathology, especially depression, anxiety disorder or eating disorder. Since the effects of coping problems and psychological disorders may be especially malevolent for people with diabetes, effective psychological treatment is especially important for these individuals. Clinicians seeking to improve metabolic and emotional outcomes for patients with diabetes should keep the following points in mind.

- The daily demands of diabetes care, the physical consequences of acute fluctuations in blood glucose level, and the reality or fear of long term diabetes complications, lead to high levels of sub-clinical, often diabetes-specific, emotional distress.[112]

- Diabetes-specific coping skill training, designed to help patients manage the myriad daily demands of life with diabetes, appears to be an effective intervention for resolving sub-clinical distress.

- Patients with diabetes also have an elevated risk for various psychological disorders, including depression, anxiety disorders and eating disorders.

- Diagnosing psychological disorders in patients with diabetes may require special care, as signs and symptoms of most common disorders may overlap with symptoms of hyperglycemia (depression), hypoglycaemia (anxiety disorders) or normal and functional attention to eating (eating disorders). Using sensitive and valid criterion-based systems such as the DSM-IV facilitates this process, since the DSM-IV does not allow symptoms attributable to a medical condition to count toward the diagnosis of a disorder.

- Psychological disorders can be especially devastating for patients with diabetes. For example, episodes of depression appear to be more frequent and severe than in the general population. In addition, all the most common disorders can interfere with diabetes management. Less active self-care may contribute to elevated blood glucose levels, increased risk of acute and long term diabetes complications and worsened quality of life.

- Research on effective treatments for psychological disorders in patients with diabetes is limited.[113] Findings to date suggest that treatments known to be effective in the general population are also effective in patients with diabetes. These treatments include (1) CBT and antidepressant medication for depression, (2) BART and anxiolytic medication for anxiety disorders and (3) standard psychotherapeutic, psychoeducational and psychopharmacologic treatments for eating disorders.

- While therapies known to be effective in the general population are probably also effective in patients with diabetes, the fact a person has diabetes should be taken into account in applying these treatments. Specific considerations include (1) side-effect profiles for certain psychotropic medications, especially anti-depressants and (2) the need to focus on diabetes-specific issues in psycho-therapy, including diabetes-specific cognitions in CBT.

- Not all emotional consequences of diabetes are negative. Many people also report positive experiences. These experiences often reflect a deepened capacity for self-awareness, self-confidence, hope and humour. Helping patients identify and reflect on such experiences can have immediate benefits as well as more enduring ones, to the degree that this facilitates motivation for self-care.

- Guidelines should be established for screening, referral and treatment of patients with diabetes and comorbid psychological problems. Psychologists and other mental health specialists should play an integral role as members of the diabetes health care team in addressing these problems.

References

1. Rubin RR, Peyrot M. Was Willis right? Thoughts on the association of depression and diabetes. *Diabetes Metabo Res Rev* 2002; **18**: 173–175.
2. Polonsky WH, Anderson Bj, Lohrer PA *et al.* Assessment of diabetes-related distress. *Diabetes Care* 1995; **18**: 754–760.
3. Egede LE, Zheng D. Independent factors associated with major depressive disorder in a national sample. *Diabetes Care* 2003; **26**: 104–111.
4. Kessler RC, Berglund P, Demler O *et al.* The epidemiology of major depressive disorder: results from the National Comorbidity Replication (NCS-R). *JAMA* 2003; **289**: 3095–3105.
5. Ciechanowski PS, Katon WJ, Russo JE. Depression and diabetes: impact of depressive symptoms on adherence, function, and costs. *Arch Intern Med* 2000; **160**: 3278–3285.
6. Lustman PJ, Anderson RJ, Freedland KE *et al.* Depression and poor glycemic control: a meta-analytic review of the literature. *Diabetes Care* 2000; **23**: 934–942.
7. de Groot M, Anderson R, Freedland KE, Clouse RE, Lustman PJ. Association of depression and diabetes complications: a meta-analysis. *Psychosom Med* 2001; **63**: 619–630.
8. Rosenthal MJ, Fajardo M, Gilmore S, Morley JE, Naliboff BD. Hospitalization and mortality of diabetes in older adults. A 3-year prospective study. *Diabetes Care* 1998, **21**: 231–235.
9. Clouse RE, Lustman PJ, Freedland KE *et al.* Depression and coronary heart disease in women with diabetes. *Psychosom Med* 2003; **65**: 376–383.
10. Egede LE, Zheng D, Simpson K. Comorbid depression is associated with increased health care use and expenditures in individuals with diabetes. *Diabetes Care* 2002; **25**: 464–470.
11. Peyrot M, Rubin R, Siminerio L. Physician and nurse use of psychosocial strategies and referrals in diabetes. *Diabetes* 2002; **51** (Suppl. 2): A446.

12. Welch GW, Jacobson AM, Polonsky WH. The Problem Areas in Diabetes Scale: an evaluation of its clinical utility. *Diabetes Care* 1997; **20**: 760–766.

13. Piette JD, Heisler M, Wagner TH. Problems paying out-of-pocket medication costs among older adults with diabetes. *Diabetes Care* 2004; **27**: 384–391.

14. Lin EH, Katon W, Vo Korff M *et al*. Relationship of depression and diabetes self-care, medication adherence, and preventive care. *Diabetes Care* 2004; **27**: 2154–2160.

15. Sommerfield AJ, Deary IJ, Frier BM. Acute hyperglycemia alters mood state and impairs cognitive performance in people with type 2 diabetes. *Diabetes Care* 2004; **27**: 2335–2340.

16. Cox D, Gonder-Frederick L, McCall A *et al*. The effects of glucose fluctuation on cognitive function and quality of life: the functional costs of hypoglycaemia among adults with type 1 or type 2 diabetes. *Int J Clin Pract* 2002; **129**: 20–26.

17. Van der Does FE, De Neeling JN, Snoek FJ *et al*. Symptoms and well-being in relation to glycemic control in type II diabetes. *Diabetes Care* 1996; **19**: 204–210.

18. Lau C, Qureshi AK, Scott SG. Association between glycaemic control and quality of life in diabetes mellitus. *J Postgrad Med* 2004; **50**: 189–194.

19. Rubin RR, Peyrot M. Quality of life and diabetes. *Diabetes/Metab Res Rev* 1999; **15**: 205–218.

20. Irvine AA, Cox D, Goner-Frederick L. Fear of hypoglycemia: relationship to physical and psychological symptoms of patients with insulin-dependent diabetes mellitus. *Health Psychol* 1992; **11**: 135–138.

21. Rubin RR. Hypoglycemia and quality of life. *Can J Diabetes Care* 2002; **26**: 60–63.

22. Peyrot M, Matthews D, Snoek F *et al*. An international study of psychological resistance to insulin use among persons with diabetes. *Diabetologia* 2003; **46** (Suppl. 1): A89.

23. Peyrot M. Psychological insulin resistance: overcoming barriers to insulin therapy. *Pract Diabetol* 2004; **23**: 6–12.

24. Korytkowski M. When oral agents fail: practical barriers to starting insulin. *Int J Obes Relat Metab Disord* 2002; **26** (Suppl 3): S18–S24.

25. Follansbee DJ, La Greca AM, Citrin WS. Coping skills training for adolescents with diabetes. *Diabetes* 1983; **32** (Suppl. 1): 37A.

26. Boardway RH, Delameter AM, Tomankowsky J *et al*. Stress management training for adolescents with diabetes. *J Pediatr Psychol* 1993: **18**: 29–45.

27. Gross AM, Heimann I, Shapiro R *et al*. Children with diabetes: social skills training and hemoglobin A1c levels. *Behav Modification* 1983: **7**: 151–164.

28. Smith KE, Schreiner BJ, Brouhard BH *et al*. Impact of camp experience on choice of coping strategies for adolescents with insulin-dependent diabetes mellitus. *Diabetes Educ* 1991: **17**: 49–53.

29. Chawick MW, Kaplan RM, Schimmel LE. Social learning intervention improves metabolic control in type 1 diabetic teenagers. *Diabetes* 1984; **33** (Suppl. 1): 69A.

30. Mendez FJ, Melendez M. Effects of a behavioral intervention on treatment adherence and stress management in adolescents with IDDM. *Diabetes Care* 1997; **20**: 1370–1375.

31. Shalom R, Ryan J. Support and education groups for type 1 diabetics in a college campus. *Diabetes* 1987; **36** (Suppl. 1): 210A.

32. Grey M, Boland EA, Davidson M *et al*. Short-term effects of coping skills training as an adjunct to intensive therapy in adolescents. *Diabetes Care* 1998; **21**: 902–908.

33. Grey M, Boland EA, Davidson M, Tamborlane WV. Coping skills training for youth with diabetes mellitus has long-lasting effects on metabolic control and quality of life. *J Pediatr* 2000; **137**: 107–113.

34. Wysocki T, Greco P, Harris MA *et al*. Behavior therapy for families of adolescents with diabetes: maintenance of treatment effects. *Diabetes Care* 2001; **24**: 441–446.

35. Sandor J. The effect of diabetic camp on locus of control. *Diabetes* 1981; **30** (Suppl. 1): 49A.

36. Moffatt MEK, Pless IB. Locus of control in juvenile diabetic campers. *J Pediatr* 1983; **103**: 146–150.
37. Scharf LS, Leach DC, Adams KM. Diabetes camp as a psychological intervention. *Diabetes* 1987; **36** (Suppl. 1): 109A.
38. McCraw RK, Travis LB. Psychological effects of a special summer camp on juvenile diabetics. *Diabetes* 1973; **22**: 275–278.
39. Marrero DG, Meyers GI, Golden MP *et al*. Adjustment to misfortune: the use of a social support group for adolescents with diabetes. *Pediatr Adolesc Endocrinol* 1982; **10**: 213–218.
40. Anderson BJ, Wolf, FM, Burkhart MT *et al*. Effects of peer-group interventions on metabolic control in adolescents with IDDM: randomized outpatient study. *Diabetes Care* 1989; **12**: 179–183.
41. Karlsen B, Idsoe T, Dirdal I *et al*. Effects of a group-based counseling programme on diabetes-related stress, coping, psychological well-being and metabolic control in adults with type 1 or type 2 diabetes. *Patient Educ Couns* 2004; **53**: 299–308.
42. Pibernik-Okanovic M, Prasek M, Poljicanin-Filipovic T *et al*. Effects of an empowerment-based psychosocial intervention on quality of life and metabolic control in type 2 diabetic patients. *Patient Educ Couns* 2004; **52**: 193–199.
43. Warren-Boulton E, Anderson BJ, Schwartz NL *et al*. A group approach to the management of diabetes in adolescents and young adults. *Diabetes Care* 1981; **4**: 620–623.
44. Dupois A. Assessment of the psychological factors and responses in self-managed patients. *Diabetes Care* 1980; **3**: 117–120.
45. Rabin C, Amir S, Nardi R *et al*. Compliance and control issues in group training for diabetics. *Health Soc Work* 1986; **11**: 141–151.
46. Cain C, Childs C. Development of a peer support group for patients using a subcutaneous insulin infusion pump. *Diabetes* 1982; **31** (Suppl. 1): 18A.
47. Aveline MO, McCulloch DK, Tattersall RB. The practice of group psychotherapy with adult insulin-dependent diabetics. *Diab Med* 1985; **2**: 275–282.
48. American Diabetes Association. National standards for diabetes self-management education. *Diabetes Care* 2000; **23**: 682–689.
49. Peyrot M, Rubin RR. Living with diabetes: the patient-centered perspective. *Diabetes Spectrum* 1994; **7**: 204–205.
50. Rubin RR, Biermann J, Toohey B. *Psyching Out Diabetes: a Positive Approach to Your Negative Emotions*, 3rd ed. Los Angeles: Lowell House, 1999.
51. Rubin RR, Peyrot M, Saudek CD. The effect of a diabetes education program incorporating coping skills training on emotional well-being and diabetes self efficacy. *The Diabetes Educator* 1993; **19**: 210–214.
52. Rubin RR, Walen S, Ellis A. Living with diabetes: a rational–emotive therapy perspective. *J Rational-Emotive Cognitive–Behavioral Ther* 1990; **8**: 21–39.
53. Marlatt GA, Gordon JR. *Relapse Prevention: a Self-Control Strategy for the Maintenance of Behavior Change*. New York: Guilford, 1985.
54. Rubin RR, Peyrot M, Saudek CD. Effect of diabetes education on self-care, metabolic control, and emotional well-being. *Diabetes Care* 1989; **12**: 673–679.
55. Rubin RR, Peyrot M, Saudek CD. Differential effect of diabetes education on self-regulation and lifestyle behaviors. *Diabetes Care* 1991; **14**: 335–338.
56. Peyrot M, Rubin RR. Modeling the effect of diabetes education on glycemic control. *Diabetes Educator* 1994; **20**: 143–148.
57. Peyrot M, Rubin RR. Structure and correlates of diabetes-specific locus of control. *Diabetes Care* 1994; **17**: 994–1001.

58. Peyrot M, Rubin RR. Persistence of depressive symptoms in diabetes. *Diabetes Care* 1999; **22**: 448–452.

59. Peyrot M, McMurry JF. Stress-buffering and glycemic control: the role of coping styles. *Diabetes Care* 1992; **15**: 842–846.

60. Peyrot M, McMurry JF, Kruger DF. A biopsychosocial model of glycemic control in diabetes: stress, coping and regimen adherence. *J Health Soc Behav* 1999; **40**: 141–158.

61. Gavard JA, Lustman PJ, Clouse RE. Prevalence of depression in adults with diabetes: an epidemiological evaluation. *Diabetes Care* 1993; **16**: 1167–1178.

62. Grigsby AB, Anderson RJ, Freedland KE *et al*. Prevalence of anxiety in adults with diabetes: a systematic review. *J Psychosom Res* 2002; **53**: 1053–1060.

63. Colton P, Olmsted M, Daneman D *et al*. Disturbed eating behavior and eating disorders in preteen and early teenage girls with type 1 diabetes: a case-controlled study. *Diabetes Care* 2004; **27**: 1654–1659.

64. Grylli V, Hafferl-Gattermayer A, Schober E, Karwautz A. Prevalence and manifestations of eating disorders in Austrian adolescents with type 1 diabetes. *Wein Klin Wochenscchr* 2004; **116**: 230–234.

65. Goodwin RD, Hoven CW, Spitzer RL. Diabetes and eating disorders in primary care. *Int J Eat Disord* 2003; **33**: 85–91.

66. Svensson M, Engstrom I, Aman J. Higher drive for thinness in adolescent males with insulin-dependent diabetes mellitus compared with healthy controls. *Acta Paediatr* 2003; **92**: 114–117.

67. Rydall AC, Rodin GM, Olmsted MP *et al*. Disordered eating behavior and microvascular complications in young women with insulin-dependent diabetes mellitus. *N Engl J Med* 1997; **336**: 1849–1854.

68. De Berardis G, Pellegrini F, Franciosi M *et al*. Identifying patients with type 2 diabetes with higher likelihood of erectile dysfunction: the role of the interaction between clinical and psychological factors. *J Urol* 2003; **169**: 422–428.

69. American Psychiatric Association. *Diagnostic and Statistical Manual of Mental Disorders* Washington, DC: American Psychiatric Association, 1994, p 327.

70. Ciechanowski PS, Katon WJ, Russo JE, Hirsch IB. The relationship of depressive symptoms to symptom reporting, self-care and glucose control in diabetes. *Gen Hosp Psychiatry* 2003; **25**: 246–252.

71. Lustman PJ, Harper GW. Nonpsychiatric physicians' identification of depression in patients with diabetes. *Compr Psychiatry* 1987; **28**: 22–27.

72. Spitzer RL, Kroenke K, Williams JBW *et al*. Validation and utility of a self-report version of the PRIME-MD: the PHQ Primary Care Study. *JAMA* 1999; **282**: 1737–1744.

73. Beck AT, Beamesderfer A. Assessment of depression: the Depression Inventory. *Med Probl Psychopharmacother* 1974; **7**: 151–169.

74. Radloff LS. The CES-D scale: a self-report depression scale for research in the general population. *Appl Psych Meas* 1977; **3**: 385–401.

75. Henkel V, Mergl R, Coyne JC *et al*. Screening for depression in primary care: will one or two items suffice? *Eur Arch Psychiatry Clin Neurosci* 2004; **254**: 215–223.

76. Henkel V, Mergl R, Kohnen R *et al*. Use of brief depression screening tools in primary care: consideration of heterogeneity in performance in different patient groups. *Gen Hosp Psychiatry* 2004; **26**: 190–198.

77. Bonsignore M, Barkow K, Jessen F, Heun R. Validity of the five-item WHO Well-Being Index (WHO-5) in an elderly population. *Eur Arch Psychiatry Clin Neurosci* 2001; **251** (Suppl. 2): II27–II31.

78. Lustman PJ, Griffith LS, Clouse RE *et al.* Effects of nortriptyline on depression and glycemic control in diabetes: results of a double-blind, placebo-controlled trial. *Psychosom Med* 1997; **59**: 241–250.

79. Lustman PJ, Freedland KE, Griffith LS, Clouse RE. Fluoxetine for depression in diabetes: a randomized, double-blind, placebo-controlled trial. *Diabetes Care* 2000; **23**: 618–623.

80. Lustman PJ, Griffith LS, Freedland KE *et al.* Cognitive behavior therapy for depression in type 2 diabetes: a randomized controlled trial. *Ann Intern Med* 1998; **129**: 613–621.

81. Williams JW, Katon WJ, Lin EHB *et al.* The effectiveness of depression care management on diabetes-related outcomes in older patients. *Ann Intern Med* 2004; **140**: 1015–1024.

82. Katon WJ, Von Korff M, Lin EHB *et al.* The Pathways study: a randomized trial of collaborative care in patients with diabetes and depression. *Arch Gen Psychiatry* 2004; **61**: 1042–1049.

83. Rubin RR, Ciechanowski P, Egede LE, Lin EHB, Lustman P. Recognizing and treating depression in patients with diabetes. *Curr Diabetes Rep* 2004; **4**: 119–125.

84. Lustman PJ, Griffith LS, Clouse RE. Depression in adults with diabetes: results of a 5-year follow-up study. *Diabetes Care* 1988; **11**: 605–612.

85. Popkin MK, Callies AL, Lentz RD *et al.* Prevalence of major depression, simple phobia, and other psychiatric disorders in patients with long-standing type 1 diabetes mellitus. *Arch Gen Psychiatry* 1988; **45**: 64–68.

86. Thomas J, Jones G, Scarini I, Brantley P. A descriptive and comparative study of depressive and anxiety disorders in low-income adults with type 2 diabetes and other chronic illnesses. *Diabetes Care* 2003; **26**: 2311–2317.

87. Kruse J, Schmitz N, Thefeld W. On the association between diabetes and mental disorders in a community sample: results from the German national Health Interview and Examination Survey. *Diabetes Care* 2003; **26**: 1841–1846.

88. Peyrot M, Rubin RR. Levels and risks of depression and anxiety symptomatology among diabetic adults. *Diabetes Care* 1997; **20**: 585–590.

89. McGrady A, Bailey BK, Good MP. Controlled study of biofeedback-assisted relaxation in type I diabetes. *Diabetes Care* 1991; **14**: 360–365.

90. Zettler A, Duran G, Waadt S *et al.* Coping with fear of long-term complications in diabetes mellitus: a model clinical program. *Psychother Psychosom* 1995; **64**: 178–184.

91. Okada S, Ichiki K, Tanokuchi S *et al.* Effects of an anxiolytic on lipid profile in non-insulin-dependent diabetes mellitus. *J Intern Med Res* 1994; **22**: 338–342.

92. Lustman PJ, Griffith LS, Clouse RE *et al.* Effects of alprazolam on glucose regulation in diabetes. *Diabetes Care* 1995; **18**: 1133–1139.

93. Hall RCW. Bulimia nervosa and diabetes mellitus. *Semin Clin Neuropsychiatry* 1997; **2**: 24–30.

94. Kenardy J, Mensch M, Bown K *et al.* Disordered eating behaviours in women with type 2 diabetes mellitus. *Eat Behav* 2001; **2**: 183–192.

95. Crow S, Kendall D, Praus B, Thuras P. Binge eating and other psychopathology in patients with type II diabetes mellitus. *Int J Eat Disord* 2001; **30**: 222–226.

96. Hepertz S, Albus C, Lichtblau K *et al.* Relationship of weight and eating disorders in type 2 diabetic patients: a multicenter study. *Int J Eat Disord* 2000; **28**: 68–77.

97. Mannucci E, Tesi F, Rica V *et al.* Eating behavior in obese patients with and without type 2 diabetes mellitus. *Int J Obes Relat Metab Disord* 2002; **26**: 848–853.

98. LaGreca A, Schwartz L, Satin W *et al.* Binge eating among women with IDDM: associations with weight dissatisfaction, adherence, and metabolic control. *Diabetes* 1990; **39** (Suppl. 1): 164A.

99. Stancin T, Link DL, Reuter JM. Binge eating in young women with IDDM. *Diabetes Care* 1989; **12**: 601–603.

100. Wing RR, Norwalk MP, Marcus MD *et al.* Subclinical eating disorders and glycemic control in adolescents with type 1 diabetes. *Diabetes Care* 1986; **9**: 162–167.
101. Steel JM, Young RJ, Lloyd GG, Clarke BF. Clinically apparent eating disorders in young diabetic women: association with painful neuropathy and other complications. *BMJ* 1987; **294**: 859–862.
102. Nielsen S, Emborg C, Molbak AG. Mortality in concurrent type 1 diabetes and anorexia nervosa. *Diabetes Care* 2002; **25**: 309–312.
103. LaGreca A, Schwartz L, Satin W. Eating patterns in young women with IDDM: another look. *Diabetes Care* 1987; **10**: 659–660.
104. Biggs MM, Basco MR, Patterson G, Raskin P. Insulin withholding for weight control in women with diabetes. *Diabetes Care* 1994; **17**: 1186–1189.
105. Polonsky WH, Anderson BJ, Lohrer P *et al.* Insulin omission in women with IDDM. *Diabetes Care* 1994; **17**: 1179–1184.
106. Pollock M, Kovacs M, Charron-Prochownik, D. Eating disorders and maladaptive dietary/ insulin management among youths with childhood-onset insulin-dependent diabetes mellitus. *J Am Acad Child Adolesc Psychiatry* 1995; **34**: 291–296.
107. Schade DS, Drumm DA, Duckworth WC, Eaton RP. The etiology of incapacitating, brittle diabetes. *Diabetes Care* 1985; **8**: 12–20.
108. Peveler RC, Fairburn CG. Anorexia nervosa in association with diabetes mellitus–a cognitive–behavioural approach to treatment. *Behav Res Ther* 1989; **27**: 95–99.
109. Rapaport WS, LaGreca AM, Levine P. Preventing eating disorders in young women with type I diabetes. In Anderson BJ, Rubin RR (eds), *Practical Psychology for Diabetes Clinicians: How to Deal With the Key Behavioral Issues Faced by Patients and Health-Care Teams* Alexandria, VA: American Diabetes Association, 1996; pp 133–142.
110. Rubin RR, Peyrot M. Psychological problems and interventions in diabetes: a review of the literature. *Diabetes Care* 1992; **15**: 1640–1657.
111. Saudek CD, Rubin RR, Shump CS. *The Johns Hopkins Guide to Diabetes.* Baltimore, MD: Johns Hopkins University Press, 1997.
112. Rubin RR, Peyrot M. Psychological issues and treatments for people with diabetes. *J Clin Psychol* 2001; **57**: 457–478.
113. Snoek FJ, Skinner TC. Psychological counselling in problematic diabetes: does it help? *Diab Med* 2002; **19**: 265–273.

Index

Psychology in Diabetes Care   Edited by Frank J. Snoek and T. Chas Skinner
© 2005 John Wiley & Sons, Ltd.

Index compiled by Christine Boylan